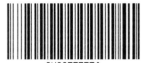

CW00555556

LOWER YOUR BLOOD PRI

★ eat a healthy, balanced d
★ take gentle exercise
★ learn to relax
★ find the right therapy for you

By the same author

CYSTITIS
DEPRESSION
HEALING POWER OF HYPNOTISM (with David Shreeve)
HEALTHY HEART FOR LIFE
PREMENSTRUAL SYNDROME

LOWER YOUR BLOOD PRESSURE

IN 4 EASY STAGES

*Natural, safe
ways to
reduce it*

Dr Caroline M. Shreeve
MB, BS (Lond)

THORSONS PUBLISHING GROUP

First published 1989

To John Poncia with lots of love

Copyright © Caroline M. Shreeve 1989

All rights reserved. No part of this book may be reproduced or utilized in any form or by any means, electronic or mechanical, including photocopying, recording or by any information storage and retrieval system, without permission in writing from the Publisher.

British Library Cataloguing in Publication Data

Shreeve, Caroline
Lower your blood pressure in 4 easy stages: natural, safe
ways to reduce it.
1. Man. Blood. Hypertension. Therapy
I. Title
616.1'3206

ISBN 0 7225 1635 5

Published by Thorsons Publishers Limited, Wellingborough, Northamptonshire NN8 2RQ, England

Typeset by Harper Phototypesetters Limited, Northampton, England
Printed in Great Britain by Mackays of Chatham, Kent

10 9 8 7 6 5 4

Contents

Introduction 7

Part One: Diagnosing high blood pressure 9

1 Problems with orthodox treatments 11
Antihypertensive drugs and their side-effects
Less common drugs
Practical problems
Progress report

2 What *is* blood pressure? 23
How the blood circulates
How blood pressure is measured
Defining hypertension
The causes
Risk factors

3 Hypertension and health problems 37
Heart failure
Kidney failure
Strokes
Atherosclerosis
Coronary heart disease

4 The treatment controversy 47
Research
Women and hypertension
The elderly and hypertension
Choice of medication
Patients, doctors and medication

Part Two: Reducing your blood pressure naturally   57

5 Diet and weight control   59
Diet: its aims
Improved health and vitality diet
Eating to reduce high blood pressure
Eating to lower a blood fat level
Weight reduction

6 Helpful dietary supplements   76
Malnutrition in the West
Supplements for high blood pressure and the circulation
Anti-stress supplements
Weight reduction nutrients

7 Easy exercise   87
The effects of exercise
Benefits of exercise
How to start

8 Relaxation techniques   96
Harnessing parasympathetic power

9 Cigarettes, alcohol and hypertension   104
Cigarettes and your body
Cigarette smoking — how to stop
Alcohol and high blood pressure
Alcohol and your body
What constitutes abuse?
Who is at risk?
How to stop drinking

10 Alternative therapies   113
Naturopathy
Herbal medicine
Homoeopathy
Acupuncture
Useful addresses

Index   125

Introduction

Yes you *can* reduce your blood pressure naturally and safely! Proven self-help methods can often reduce a mildly or moderately raised blood pressure unaided, or enable your doctor to prescribe lower doses of drugs should these remain necessary.

Claims to cure 'blood pressure' overnight have been made in the past by catch-penny charlatans whose miracle remedies turn out to be a disappointing waste of money. You will find no claims for miracle cures in this book. The information it contains is based upon the results of scientific studies and upon the established usefulness of a number of complementary (i.e. alternative) therapies.

If you are in your twenties or thirties and have — so far as you know — perfectly normal blood pressure, you may think of hypertension (abnormally raised blood pressure) as a complaint of older people. Certainly the average blood pressure in Western countries does rise with age; but far from being normal, this is a reflection of our lifestyle and a major risk factor in the development of heart and arterial disease.

Recent research has shown that the blood pressure readings of some 'healthy' teenagers equal those of many middle-aged adults. Hypertension produces few if any symptoms in its early stages, so take the precaution of having your blood pressure checked every six months. Follow the lifestyle hints in this book to keep your blood pressure within acceptable limits, and improve your vitality and well-being.

If you are already a sufferer, the combination of a healthier lifestyle and natural remedies will help to relieve your disorder and increase your capacity to live a fuller, longer, and more enjoyable life.

PART ONE:

Diagnosing high blood pressure

CHAPTER 1

Problems with orthodox treatments

Awareness of high blood pressure is vital. Some doctors feel that a mildly raised blood pressure need not be treated with drugs, providing a careful eye is kept upon the patient's progress. Advice is usually given about appropriate lifestyle changes, such as losing excess weight. Seriously raised blood pressure is a grave condition, leading to life-threatening disorders which will be examined in detail in Chapter 3.

Antihypertensive drugs have been the mainstay of medical treatment since they first became available in 1950, and they have extended and improved the quality of life for millions of people. Details of how they work can be found in Chapter 4. Like other drugs, though, they are capable of causing side-effects, which in some cases can be severe. At all times, the extent to which blood pressure can be reduced to normal or near-normal levels has to be determined in part by the likelihood of causing adverse reactions. One of the reasons that 11 main classes of antihypertensive drugs have been produced is to make the choice of acceptable treatment as wide as possible.

If you are a sufferer, the chances are that you see your GP every month or so, have your blood pressure checked, and receive another prescription for tablets — simple 'water pills', or beta blockers alone or in combination with water pills (discussed later in this chapter), or one of the other drugs now available. Your doctor may advise you to lose weight, change your diet, give up smoking, or relax more often. Lifestyle habits that require self-denial and willpower to alter, though, often remain fixed — especially if we are unconvinced that changing them will really be worth the effort.

I urge all readers to take such advice to heart, and to follow it implicitly. The entrenched image of doctors — especially of GPs — as animated, prescription-writing robots is rapidly becoming outdated. Orthodox and alternative medicine are no longer poles apart, and as the two have warily approached one another after the initial 'territorial' snarling period, each has benefited from the other's philosophy.

Alternative therapists — medical herbalists, acupuncturists, osteopaths, aromatherapists — have accepted the need to provide, if not a strictly scientific explanation for their treatments, at least acceptable evidence that they work. Orthodox doctors, on the other hand, are starting to accept the essential principle of holistic theory of a person as a whole being, and to recognize mental and spiritual needs as well as those of the body. Thanks to the influence of complementary medicine, the viewing of a patient as a set of interesting symptoms indicative of a particular pathology is now regarded as inadequate.

One result of this is the growing acceptance of effective drug-free remedies by orthodox doctors. During the past five years, there has been immense interest among cardiovascular (heart and blood circulation) specialists and research scientists in the use of natural methods of blood pressure control as alternatives or adjuncts to standard drug therapy. The question of whether patients with mild, symptomless raised blood pressure really require treatment has been debated for some time; and, increasingly, patients who need therapy are being encouraged to put self-help treatment methods into practice.

In this context, we must also remember the more mundane influence of the cost of prescribing expensive drugs over long periods, and the time required to see patients in overtaxed surgeries and out-patient clinics. A GP with a list size of 2,500 patients can expect to have 375 patients with raised blood pressure to assess and manage.

The questions of how 'normal' and 'high' blood pressure are defined, how high a particular patient's blood pressure can rise before it requires treatment, and the means by which the various antihypertensive drugs work will be looked at in Chapters 3 and 4. Here, we will take a look at some of their side-effects, and the practical problems connected with their use. The idea is not to dissuade you from taking them, but to enable you to relate adverse reactions, should they arise, to your medication, and not to misconstrue them as some mysterious ailment.

It's important to remember that most problems related to drugs settle down and disappear with time, and that many people take them for years wihout encountering side-effects of any sort. Consult your doctor if you find your tablets or capsules do not suit you. It is very unwise to stop taking drugs of your own accord, especially those for high blood pressure. It is often a simple matter to change the prescription to something more suitable, should this prove necessary.

Because it is customary for hypertensive patients to remain on drugs for a considerable time, sometimes permanently, their side-effects have generated many research studies and the consequent development of safer and more effective compounds. They have also led to increased interest in drug-free treatment methods among health experts of both orthodox and complementary disciplines.

Antihypertensive drugs and their side-effects

Diuretics

Diuretics ('water pills') make you pass more urine than usual. This is how they reduce blood pressure, so it can hardly be called a side-effect! All the same, the need to visit the toilet frequently can pose serious problems to many people (see Practical problems, later in this chapter). Generally, though, a diuretic producing a gradually increasing water loss is chosen in preference to one whose brief, dramatic effect keeps you rushing to the toilet for two or three hours.

Although these drugs are acceptable to most people, some can cause loss of potassium in the urine and make you tired, weak and drowsy, and may cause an irregular heart beat (*arrhythmia*) if a serious deficiency develops. This is especially likely to happen to elderly people who frequently eat insufficient potassium-rich foods such as meat, milk and milk products, fresh vegetables (especially the green, leafy type) and fruit.

Diuretics can also cause nausea and diarrhoea, faintness, pins and needles, cramps, and itchy rashes. Men taking them may have difficulty in sustaining an erection. Many increase the blood fat (cholesterol) level, a major factor in the development of clogged arteries (see Atherosclerosis, Chapter 3), and affect uric acid metabolism, increasing the risk of gout. Being seriously overweight predisposes you to a high blood sugar and diabetes, and these may be aggravated by diuretics, which is yet another incentive for you to shed surplus pounds.

Examples of diuretics include frusemide — furosemide in the USA — (Lasix, Frusene, Frusetic, Aluzine); triamterene (Frusene, Dytzac, Dytide); and the thiazide group, such as bendrofluazide (Aprinox, Berkozide, Inderetic, Neo-naclex).

Beta blockers

Some people taking 'beta blocker' drugs also get tummy upsets and skin rashes, a slow pulse, cold hands and feet, and sleep disturbed by vivid dreams. Cold hands are a particular problem in elderly people, who are also less able to cope with the drowsiness, confusion and poor sleep that can result.

Like diuretics, beta blockers can worsen blood sugar control in some diabetics on insulin or drugs such as glibenclamide (Malix, Calabren, Euglucon) or chloropropamide (Diabinese). They reduce the 'helpful', high-density variety of cholesterol known to help combat arterial disease, and can cause air tube spasm. They have to be prescribed with caution for wheezy or asthmatic patients and, for more complex reasons, for people suffering from heart failure.

Some people on beta blocker drugs may experience dryness of the eyes, although this was much more likely to happen with practolol, which is no longer available. This makes the eyes itchy and uncomfortable, and is a major nuisance if you wear contact lenses. Examples of beta blocker drugs include propranolol (Inderal, Inderetic, Apsolol); sotalol (Beta-Cardone, Sotacor, Tolerzide); and timolol (Blocadren, Moducren, Prestim, Betim).

Vasodilators

Examples of vasodilators are hydralazine (Apresoline); minoxidil (Loniten); and diazoxide (Eudemine).

Hydralazine causes a rapid heart beat (*tachycardia*), flushes, and headaches. Doses above 100mg daily can produce a condition resembling the auto-immune disease systemic lupus erythematosis, or SLE, in biologically susceptible people (mainly Caucasian women). The symptoms include skin rashes, fever, and painful joints and muscles.

Minoxidil causes rapid heart beat and tissue swelling (*oedema*) due to salt and water retention. It cannot be used to treat hypertension due to phaeochromocytoma (see Chapter 2 under Glandular causes of hypertension), and its promotion of hair growth on the face, body limbs and elsewhere makes it unsuitable for women. It is now also marketed as Regaine, a clear yellow liquid applied to the scalp to treat pattern baldness (*alopecia androgenetica*), in men only.

Diazoxide can cause nausea, high blood sugar, tremors and abnormal muscular movement. All these drugs can precipitate *angina* in patients with coronary heart disease (see Chapter 3).

Calcium antagonists

Also known as calcium channel blockers, these drugs include verapamil (Cordilox, Univer); nifedipine (Adalat and Adalat retard); and nicardipine (Cardene). Either they have no effect upon blood lipid levels, or they elevate the high density non-protective variety. Their commonest side-effects include headaches, flushes, and swelling of the toes, feet and ankles which is unrelieved by diuretic drugs.

Nifedipine can cause dizziness, lethargy, and in very rare cases hypersensitivity jaundice. Nicardipine can cause nausea, palpitations and a sensation of heat. Verapamil can cause constipation, nausea and vomiting.

Nifedipine and related compounds are incompatible in some people with Tagamet (cimetidine), a drug frequently prescribed for the treatment of peptic ulcers, as dizziness and very low blood pressure may result. When this occurs, the dose of nifedipine is either halved, or Zantac (ranitidine) substituted for the Tagamet, since it is far less likely to cause adverse reactions.

ACE inhibitors

ACE stands for 'angiotensin converting enzyme'. Examples are captopril (Capoten), enalapril (Innovace), and the recently introduced, once-daily lisinopril (Carace, Zestril).

They have fewer side-effects than many other antihypertensive drugs; those that do occur can include a sudden, dramatic fall in blood pressure (hypotension), a persistent dry cough, rashes, headaches, fatigue, dizziness, nausea and vomiting. Loss of taste (which returns to normal when the treatment stops) and angioneurotic oedema (swelling of areas of skin, mucous membranes and underlying tissue) have both been reported, but ACE inhibitors are generally well tolerated by the patients for whom they are prescribed.

Captopril can cause pruritus (itching), rashes, a cough, and mouth ulcers. Enalopril can produce muscle cramps, urticaria (nettle rash), tiredness and nausea; and lisinopril may cause lethargy, weakness, and chest pain.

Less common drugs

The drug or drugs you are taking or want to find out about may not fall within the groups just described, so here are brief notes on the other available types. The first four have been available for four years and are far less often prescribed than they once were; the final two are relative newcomers.

CNS depressants

These include: alpha-methyldopa (Aldomet, Dopamet, Medomet); clonidine (Dixarit, Catapres); and reserpine (Serpasil). The first of these was used to treat elderly hypertensive patients in a trial carried out in 1985 by Professor A. Amery and his colleagues at the University of Birmingham, and favourable results were reported in *The Lancet*. Despite this, neither it nor others in the group are often used as starting treatment for high blood pressure, but alpha-methyldopa may be used to control severe hypertension or prescribed for a patient who has been taking it for years before the consultation. Side-effects can include depression, a dry mouth and stuffy nose, drowsiness, and lethargy. Men taking these drugs occasionally experience erection problems. There have also been several reports of an increased incidence of breast cancer in middle-aged women treated with reserpine.

Adrenergic neurone blocking drugs

Examples include guanethidine (Ismelin, Ganda), debrisoquine (Declinax), and bethanidine (Esbatal, Bendogen). They were among the first antihypertensive drugs to be taken by mouth, and made a very significant contribution to hypertension therapy in the 1950s.

The side-effects limiting their use include postural hypotension (sudden fall in blood pressure on standing up, often accompanied by dizziness); failure of ejaculation; nasal stuffiness; diarrhoea and constipation.

Ganglion blockers

Ganglion blockers, e.g. trimetaphan (Arfonad), are used to treat hypertension associated with aortic aneurysm (an abnormal bulge in the side of the wall of the aorta) and are administered by intravenous injection (i.e. into a vein). Ganglion blocker side-effects include severe postural hypotension and the rapid development of tolerance (i.e. the need to give larger doses to achieve the same effect). They are usually only used during surgical procedures.

Chemoreceptor depressant drugs

Veratrum (Thiaver, Veriloid, Rauwiloid + Veriloid), the sole member of this group still available in the UK, is rarely prescribed because it tends to send the blood pressure plunging down and also to cause a high incidence of unacceptable side-effects.

Alpha blockers

Examples include prazosin (Hypovase) and indoramin (Baratol). The initial dose of prazosin may be followed by severely lowered blood pressure. Indoramin has a sedative effect and can also cause severe postural hypotensive problems. Both can cause headaches and nasal stuffiness.

Alpha-beta blockers

Labetolol (Labrocol; Trandate) is the first drug of this class to be marketed in the UK. Large doses can cause orthostatic hypotension.

Practical problems

Whether you experience side-effects from your drugs or not, it is essential to remember to take them regularly. This can be a problem if you travel frequently, have a busy daily routine, or simply have a poor memory. Opening screwtop bottles and tablet jars can be trying if you have arthritis in your hands. Container manufacturers, in their attempts to make their products childproof, seem to have forgotten that adults needing to open them may lack sufficient strength and dexterity. Even blister packs (the type in which the tablet or capsule is pushed through the metal foil backing of a card covered with clear protective wrapping) need a certain nimbleness of the fingers.

If you are elderly it is often very hard to remember to take tablets when prescribed. You may find that you have a bewildering assortment of medicines and pills of all shapes, colours, and sizes, and find that you cannot read the small, printed names and instructions on the container labels. Trying to think back to what the doctor said, while you wrestle unsuccessfully with a resistant bottle top, can cause a lot of anxiety.

Some senior citizens living alone make out lists (which it is easy to get wrong!) and set their alarm clocks to remind them that it is 'pill time' — the days seem to revolve around the next dose. If you cannot remember what the doctor said each kind was supposed to do for you, it is often tempting to forget about them and leave them to collect dust.

A better idea is to get your doctor to explain again and again, until you are certain you know exactly what you have been prescribed, and why. If your eyesight is reasonably good, then ask the doctor or the practice nurse to write the instructions down in clear handwriting or print.

The 'placebo' effect some medications can have, despite a mistaken view of what it has been prescribed for, was illustrated by tablets I once prescribed for an 80-year-old man. He thanked me profusely when he had finished the three-week course, saying that the stomach upsets, poor appetite, heartburn and hiccups which had bothered him for years had disappeared entirely. Puzzled, I consulted his notes, and found that when he had seen me earlier, he had complained of swelling and pain in his arthritic knee joints, and that in fact he had been taking the non-steroidal anti-inflammatory arthritic drug Feldene (piroxicam)!

Potassium supplements often cause confusion. These may be prescribed with certain water pills to replace reduced stores of this mineral (see above). If an elderly or confused person cannot relate them to any of his or her symptoms, then the point of taking them is not apparent.

Potassium supplements are sometimes added to the water pills themselves, removing the need for extra pill-taking. Others are supplied as a whole tablet, or as granules which make up a sparkling drink when mixed with water. However palatably they are presented, though, they often cause gut irritation and nausea.

If you suffer from bladder problems, getting to the toilet in time can be a nightmare when you are taking diuretic drugs. Public toilets seem to vanish from the earth's surface when you are out shopping and need to visit one urgently. If you are elderly or handicapped and house-bound, it can be just as difficult. Negotiating furniture and maybe long corridors in a hurry, when your walking difficulties make you frightened of falling, may result in your passing some urine before you reach your destination. This is extremely distressing, causes a lot of extra washing and ironing, and is one of the major problems of water pill treatment for anyone with limited mobility.

Among the practical difficulties you may face from the side-effects of blood pressure drugs are lethargy and drowsiness. These can affect your work, especially if you have a sedentary job in a warm, close atmosphere; or they can cause you to sleep during the daytime if you are house-bound, thus disturbing your night sleeping pattern.

Nausea, stomach pains, and diarrhoea can make you feel weak and debilitated, as well as putting you off your food; and giddy spells are especially dangerous if you drive, handle dangerous machinery, or are elderly or handicapped and alone. Headaches, stuffy nose, cold hands and feet, skin rash, poor sleep, and eye dryness can also make you miserable.

The advice that follows should help to relieve both the side-effects and the practical problems of blood pressure drugs, if you have to continue taking them in addition to the self-help methods described in this book. Reassure yourself at this point that, even if this is the case, your general health and fitness level will improve if you combine them with your medication. Indeed, you may well find that you can reduce your blood pressure satisfactorily without having to rely on prescription medicines of any kind.

Swallowing medicines

No discussion of the problems you can encounter with medication is complete without mentioning one of the commonest of them all — that of actually taking them. Many people find it difficult to swallow tablets of any type. This is most likely to be the case if you are elderly, suffer from a mouth or throat disorder, or have the type of gullet that seems to 'close up' the moment it meets a tablet or spoonful of medicine. In your experience, a spoonful of sugar is no help at all in making the medicine go down!

This problem can be partly psychological in some people, who have no problem at all in gulping half-chewed food, including hard, pill-sized pieces of salted nuts, boiled sweets or popcorn! Swallowing tablets and capsules is also difficult if you feel sick (as a result of the last dose?!), are recovering from an illness, or have a poor appetite. Dainty morsels may well slip down the 'red lane' with comparative ease, while medication leaves you gagging. Save one such treat as a reward for taking after medication, and drink plenty of water.

Progress report

You now know something of the wide variety of side-effects and practical difficulties high blood pressure sufferers may encounter with standard drug treatment. It is only fair to say that some patients experience no adverse reactions at all; and it is extremely unlikely that anyone would be affected by all the 'nasties' a particular drug is capable of causing.

If you are being treated for hypertension, you *must* remain on your course of tablets until the natural techniques you will learn about here produce a measurable improvement. It is then that your doctor will consider reducing the dose, or taking you off your tablets for a trial period. If you do experience adverse reactions to any drug, the right thing to do is to return to your GP and ask for a change of prescription to something that suits you better. Even if you have to stop taking medicines because they do not 'agree' with you, you need a substitute.

We should also acknowledge the hard work pharmaceutical scientists and doctors have put in, over the past four decades, in testing new formulae and carrying out clinical trials with a view to improving the effectiveness and acceptability of antihypertensive drug treatment. It is fashionable to criticize the pharmaceutical industries harshly for the millions of pounds they earn yearly, but it is only just, considering where we would be without adequately researched medication and innovatory pharmacological products.

The drugs containing rauwolfia alkaloids, obtained from the south-east Asian shrub *Rauwolfia serpentina*, are a case in point.

They were among the earliest of the antihypertensives to be used. Originally prescribed as sedatives, they were found to lower raised blood pressure, and the first to be prepared, reserpine (Serpasil and Serpasil Esidrex), has been used in this capacity for decades. The other rauwolfia drug is methoserpidine (Decaserpyl, Decaserpyl Plus).

These drugs act on the hormone adrenaline contained in nerves. They are prescribed far less often nowadays, which is just as well because they can cause a stuffy nose, tiredness, and diarrhoea, as well as an increased production of stomach acid (to be avoided at all costs if you have a peptic ulcer).

Another unpleasant reaction to both rauwolfia and the vasodilator drugs is postural hypotension, which makes you feel giddy and unbalanced for a few seconds on suddenly standing up, and perhaps you may even fall over. Severe depression, which in some people leads to suicidal tendencies, has also been reported in patients taking rauwolfia.

It is interesting to contrast the situation when rauwolfia compounds were the mainstay of antihypertensive treatment with the greatly improved medical facilities doctors now have at their disposal. In 1986, a report appeared in a doctors' weekly newspaper bearing the headline, 'Life expectancy boost for blood pressure victims'. It stated that medicine had scored a 'remarkable victory over malignant hypertension' (a very serious condition, see Chapters 3 and 4) 'with the possibility of near-normal life expectancy'.

The report reminded readers that 25 years earlier, the five-year survival rate in patients with retinopathy (damage to the retina of the eye due to an abnormally high blood pressure often causing blindness, and indicative of life-threatening hypertension) was less than 1 per cent. Professor John Swales and his colleagues at the Leicester hypertension clinic were now reporting five-year survival figures of 82 per cent of the first 100 patients with very serious retinopathy seen at the clinic since it began in 1974. This figure approaches the five-year survival rate for the general population of 94 per cent.

Perhaps an even more impressive outcome was mentioned in the same newspaper article, of a group of Spanish kidney specialists (diseased kidneys are a major cause of malignant hypertension) who had studied 165 affected patients between 1974 and 1984, and reported an 87 per cent five-year survival. The reduced death rate among the patients with damaged kidneys depended to a considerable extent on the early treatment of kidney failure. All the same, a great deal of the success at both centres was due to the use of drugs to control the dangerously high blood pressure, 'most patients requiring three or more drugs in combination to do so'.

The advantages of the wide range of differently acting antihypertensives, which attack the problem from a variety of angles, are clearly underlined by this report.

The same newspaper carries an interesting feature on the 'striking success' in the management of high blood pressure achieved by an open-access clinic at Stobhill General Hospital using a number of innovations. These included adequate consultation time, flexible appointments, nurses to carry out routine tests, and individual advice to patients about diet and giving up smoking.

Of the 500 patients attending the clinic, 175 had been attending for four years. Good blood pressure control had risen from 22 per cent to 79 per cent. The results were achieved primarily on a simple regimen of a beta blocker in 70 per cent of the cases, combined with a diuretic if necessary. Only one third of the patients needed a vasodilator drug as well.

Disappointingly, though (the writer added), the clinic approach had not influenced either smoking habits or weight reduction in severely overweight patients.

My point in including the last piece of information is not to imply that smoking and being overweight are not seriously harmful, particularly for hypertension sufferers, but to point out how much better even these admirable results might have been, had the patients complied with the advice they were given. Many of them would very probably have been able to keep their own blood pressure within healthy limits without the help of drugs, or at least to have their doctors reduce their medication doses.

Vital messages cannot be repeated too often; and I will say again here, that *all* cases of hypertension must be diagnosed and dealt with. Before describing the many things you can do to reduce your own blood pressure (as well as precisely how to go about them!), it is necessary to explain what blood pressure actually *is*, why it is essential to life, and how, when seriously raised, it can cause grave organ damage and death.

CHAPTER 2

What *is* blood pressure?

You must have heard people say, 'I've got blood pressure'. It is a very good job that they have, since without it they would be dead! A critically ill or injured patient rushed into hospital has his or her blood pressure checked immediately by the casualty officer or nurse, and a low or absent (i.e. unrecordable) reading indicates a state of severe shock. Restoring it to normal is a vital, life-saving procedure.

People really mean that they have a *raised* blood pressure, which can be equally life-threatening in the long term. Its potential for harm can best be understood through acquaintance with the normal circulatory pressure, the factors that regulate it, and how it can get out of control.

How the blood circulates

Our 5 litres (about a gallon) of blood are driven around the body by the heart, a two-sided pump. Blood drains into its right side from the veins and is directed to the lungs, where it gives off carbon dioxide and picks up a fresh supply of oxygen. It then enters the left side of the heart, and is recirculated around the body. En route, waste material is removed by the kidneys, and digested nutrients are picked up from the stomach and small bowel.

Blood flows from the heart to the periphery of the body in arteries. The largest of all is the *aorta*, which comes off your heart just behind the top of your breast bone, giving off big supply branches to your neck and arms. It then runs down inside your chest and abdomen in front of your backbone, giving off further branches, and finally divides in your pelvis into the right and left femoral arteries that supply blood to your legs.

This system is like a road map, with the aorta as the motorway, giving off 'A-road' arteries to important towns. You can easily locate these by feeling your pulse at various points. The large brachial artery in your arm produces a 'thrust' on the inside of your elbow joint.

The carotid arteries running up your throat can be found pounding away an inch or so on either side of your Adam's apple. If you get frightened or excited and your heart starts to race, you usually become aware of their throb. Unless you are very fat, their pulse can be seen below the surface of your skin, and helps to give the game away about how you are reacting!

If you feel deep within your groin with your finger tips (don't dig too hard!), you will feel your femoral artery, the source of supply to your thigh and calf muscles, your feet and toes.

All these 'A-road' arteries give off smaller 'B-roads' to the various organs and muscles between which they pass. They, in turn, divide into even smaller ones, ending up as little unclassified roadways, the arterioles, which finally divide into the tiniest of all the vessels, the capillaries. These form a vast network of minute footpaths and bridle tracks with a diameter of about $\frac{1}{100}$ millimetre (0.01mm) and run through the tissues themselves.

Blood delivered to the capillaries by the arterioles is rich in oxygen and essential nutrients (e.g. glucose, amino acids). These pass out through the capillary walls into the surrounding tissue fluid and so to the cells. Under normal conditions, large protein molecules and blood cells remain within, although the white cells are capable of getting through when they need to. When injury or invading bacteria cause inflammation, histamine is secreted by the damaged cells and the walls of the capillaries leak. Extra fluid from the plasma, white cells, and occasionally red cells then escape into the surrounding tissue spaces.

As oxygen and nutrients pass out of the capillaries, carbon dioxide and other waste products of cellular metabolism pass in. The capillaries link up with small veins (venules) which join to form larger and larger vessels on the way back to the heart and lungs. In this way, capillaries are both the end of the arterial system and the start of the venous (vein) system, and form a vital bridge between the two.

The discovery of the capillaries was made by Marcello Malpighi, seventeenth century professor of medicine and

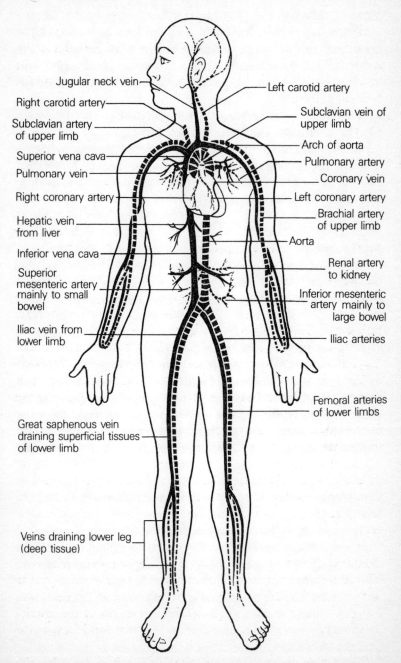

Jugular neck vein

Right carotid artery

Subclavian artery of upper limb

Superior vena cava

Pulmonary vein

Right coronary artery

Hepatic vein from liver

Inferior vena cava

Superior mesenteric artery mainly to small bowel

Iliac vein from lower limb

Great saphenous vein draining superficial tissues of lower limb

Veins draining lower leg (deep tissue)

Left carotid artery

Subclavian vein of upper limb

Arch of aorta

Pulmonary artery

Coronary vein

Left coronary artery

Brachial artery of upper limb

Aorta

Renal artery to kidney

Inferior mesenteric artery mainly to large bowel

Iliac arteries

Femoral arteries of lower limbs

Fig. 1 Circulatory system

anatomy at Bologna and Pisa, and the first professional anatomist to work with a microscope. Malpighi's breakthrough was a highly important extension of William Harvey's discovery of the circulation of the blood in 1628. Harvey realized that blood travelled continuously around the body but, having to base his observation and deductions entirely upon what he could observe with the naked eye, he could not identify the means by which blood passed from the arteries to the veins.

Harvey's findings marked the end of the era of ancient medicine and the beginning of modern medical science. Malpighi's contribution set the scene for a vast increase in our understanding of anatomy, physiology, and cellular metabolism.

The nature of blood pressure

In a healthy person, the pressure of the blood leaving the heart is around 120 mm of mercury, i.e. 2.4 lb per square inch. Because the motorway and A-road arteries are wide, the flow of blood within them meets little resistance, and its pressure is largely unaltered. The arm artery is chosen for measuring its value, both for this reason and because it is easily accessible to the doctor's blood pressure cuff and stethoscope.

The B-road branches are narrower, but there are enough of them to prevent a 'traffic hold-up' of blood in the A-roads that give rise to them. However, the pressure of the blood falls progressively as the routes get more and more narrow, and the arterioles offer the greatest resistance to its flow. By the time it reaches the capillaries, it measures only about 32 mm mercury. Because the capillaries are so minute, they might be expected to offer the greatest resistance of all; but there are so many of them that they offer less than the arterioles. The drop in pressure across the capillary network is only around 20 mm mercury.

The pressure in the veins is practically nil, i.e. it is about equal to atmospheric pressure. Blood from the lower half of the body would be unable to overcome the pull of gravity and reach the heart if it were not for a number of special help factors.

One of these is the massaging effect of surrounding muscles — especially important in the veins of the legs, whose valves play an important part in preventing backflow. Another is the increase in negative pressure that develops within the chest cavity as we inhale and encourages the flow of blood along the veins in the direction of the heart.

Why we need blood pressure

The function of blood pressure is to maintain a flow of blood to every part of the body, most importantly the brain. Unlike other organs, its needs never vary, and they remain at around 750 ml of freshly oxygenated blood per minute, regardless of whether we are sleeping or waking, working or relaxing.

Temporary interference with the brain's supply, e.g. when blood pools in the legs during a long period of standing still, causes a fainting attack. Consciousness is soon regained as the person falls to the ground or places the head between the knees, since either action restores the brain's blood and oxygen supply.

A cardiac arrest, however, is a state of the greatest emergency requiring immediate resuscitative measures. When the heart ceases to beat, the circulation of the blood comes to an abrupt halt and the blood pressure falls to zero. Irreversible brain cell damage and death occur if oxygen is lacking for only three minutes.

While abnormally low blood pressure causes uncomfortable symptoms and can be fatal when extreme, significantly raised blood pressure strains the heart and blood vessels, can cause serious damage to other organs, and greatly increases the risk of heart attack, strokes and other disorders. It is therefore very important to identify high blood pressure (hypertension) in its early stages, and prevent it from rising to a dangerous level.

How blood pressure is measured

The heart pumps the blood in spurts. With each beat, it squeezes or contracts — the phase called 'systole', pronounced *sys-tol-ee* — to eject its blood into the arterial system. This pressure, around 120 mm Hg (mercury) in a normal person, is known as the systolic pressure. The heart then relaxes — 'diastole' (*dye-as-tol-ee*) — and fills up with a fresh supply of blood.

The blood pressure is prevented from falling to zero, and the flow of blood is prevented from reaching a standstill between beats, by the elastic composition of the arteries. Their walls are stretched every time the heart beats (systole), pumping blood into them, and they rebound as it relaxes during diastole. This ensures a steady stream of blood around the circulatory system at every phase of the heart's action, and keeps the pressure during diastole at around 80 mm mercury.

The sensation of force which you feel when you take your pulse is due to the difference between systolic and diastolic pressure, and is normally around 40 mm mercury.

The blood pressure is measured by means of a sphygmomanometer, the original version of which was invented by the Italian physician Riva-Rocci in 1896. There are many sophisticated modern forms but they are all based upon the principle deduced by the original designer. Its essential components are a column of mercury in a vertical, graduated tube marked in millimetres, balanced by the air inside an inflatable arm band or cuff.

This is wrapped around the upper part of the arm above the elbow. The head of the stethoscope is placed on the brachial artery on the front of the elbow joint, with the arm fully extended. The cuff is pumped up, and the point at which the sound of the arterial pulse disappears is equal to the systolic pressure. Its value is read from the calibrated mercury tube, and is the higher of the two numbers recorded during a blood pressure reading.

The lower of the two numbers is the diastolic blood pressure reading. It is detected by the stethoscope as a characteristic sound that appears as the cuff is slowly deflated.

How blood pressure is controlled

Besides the elastic recoil of the arteries, two other factors regulate the blood pressure, namely the rate at which the blood flows, and the resistance to that flow offered by the blood and its vessels.

(1) The *flow* of the circulating blood is adapted by complex nervous and chemical means to meet prevailing demands. After a meal, the autonomic nervous system — responsible for the automatic, unconscious control of bodily functions — dilates the arteries supplying the stomach and small intestine. This brings extra blood to that area to cope with the digestive processes, and is compensated by the narrowing of arteries elsewhere in the body whose demand for blood is less immediate.

When we are threatened, frightened or angry, the stress hormone adrenaline, released by reflex action from the adrenal glands, makes the heart beat faster and diverts the blood from the skin and other areas to the limb muscles. This explains the white-faced look typical of anger or terror, and prepares us for the primitive danger reaction of flight or fight.

The flow also varies enormously according to a person's state of activity. It is usually around 5 litres a minute at rest, and may be five or six times this amount during prolonged aerobic exercise such as cross-country running when the heart is beating very rapidly.

(2) The ability of the blood flow to change so readily, in response to the body's minute-by-minute needs, emphasizes the importance of *resistance* to the flow in maintaining a stable blood pressure. The thickness (viscosity) of the blood is partly responsible, i.e. the thicker a liquid, the harder it is to pump along a narrow channel. Normally, the blood's thickness does not change, which means it is the calibre of the blood vessels themselves that is largely responsible for blood pressure regulation.

This brings us to the arterioles, which are all-important in determining whether the blood pressure remains safely within the range of normality, or whether it zooms skyward, threatening health and life. We have seen the significant part the arterioles play in lowering the pressure of the blood as it passes through them to the capillary network. Their diameters vary according to whether their muscular walls are relaxed or constricted. This is determined by impulses arising in a group of nerve cells — the vasomotor centre — located in the lowest part of the brain, and reaching their muscular walls via the autonomic nervous system.

If the heart's output of blood decreases (e.g. after a sudden haemorrhage), the consequent fall in blood pressure is counteracted, at least in part, by constriction of the arteriolar walls. When the blood flow from the heart increases, it is necessary for them to relax slightly, in order to keep the blood pressure steady.

If for any reason they fail to do so, then either the flow within them must be reduced or the pressure inside them must rise. The heart continues to maintain a steady flow of blood to meet the body's requirements, however much resistance it meets. Consequently, if the calibre of the arterioles is too narrow, it simply pumps harder to overcome the obstruction. The flow continues as normal, at the cost of the blood pressure, which consequently rises.

The kidneys also play a part in blood pressure control. They are highly dependent upon a constant supply of blood, and when this is reduced, they react by releasing an enzyme, renin. This is converted in the blood into the chemical substance angiotensin, which causes the walls of the arterioles to contract, thereby raising the blood pressure and restoring the kidneys' supply of blood.

Defining hypertension

High blood pressure is so common, and can have such serious consequences, that the term 'hypertension' might be expected to have a precise meaning. In fact, health experts have expended a great deal of effort in their search from an acceptable definition.

A wide range of blood pressure values has been obtained from human population studies. When these values are plotted as a graph, there is invariably a skew towards higher ones, but no natural or obvious break separates normality from abnormality (see Fig. 2). For this reason, the definition of hypertension remains empirical, i.e. it can only be arrived at through constant observation and experiment.

Like normal body weight, normal blood pressure has come to be recognized as that which is statistically associated with the

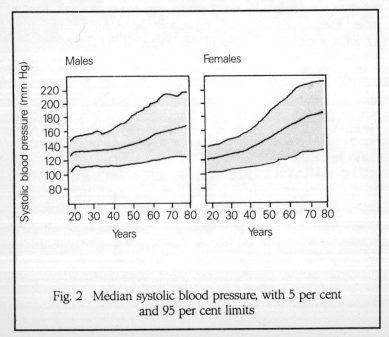

Fig. 2   Median systolic blood pressure, with 5 per cent and 95 per cent limits

greatest life expectancy. It is the level at which the heart and circulatory system are best able to carry out their work, and at which the risk of developing heart disease and other related disorders is lowest.

The systolic blood pressure may rise by as much as 50 per cent in healthy people when the blood flow increases in response to extreme emotional excitement or very vigorous exercise. It quickly returns to its resting level, however, and the diastolic pressure remains more or less unaltered throughout. The latter is the more important of the two. It reflects the condition of the arterioles, and an abnormally high reading means that they are constricted, their narrower than normal interior channels offering increased resistance to the flow of blood within them.

Mild hypertension has been variably defined in several recent treatment trials; a composite of these, providing a working definition, is a diastolic pressure of 95 to 105 mm mercury. Moderate hypertension is defined as pressure between 105 and 120, and severe hypertension above 120.

People with blood pressure of 170/110 mm mercury and above frequently experience symptoms, such as morning headaches, fatigue, and dizzy spells; and those with values above 230/130 mm mercury are highly likely to develop heart failure or other serious conditions. The greatest risk to anyone with a significantly raised blood pressure is the sudden and apparently unpredictable catastrophe of a heart attack or a stroke.

Hypertension is not a disease in the usual sense of the word, but it is the most important criterion by which doctors can predict the likelihood of future heart or circulatory disorders. It is also a risk factor that can be controlled both by antihypertensive drugs and by self-help methods.

The causes

Specific causes of hypertension can be found in only 5-10 per cent of patients. This means that they are all relatively rare but details are included here for the sake of any blood pressure sufferers who may have had one of them diagnosed.

(1) *Chronic renal disease* causes the blood pressure to rise. It damages the blood vessels of the kidneys and reduces their blood flow. This results in the release of the hormone renin (see above)

and constriction of the arterioles. Stenosis (narrowing) of the renal arteries also causes hypertension.

(2) *Glandular causes* include thyrotoxicosis (overactivity of the thyroid gland); and malfunction of the outer shell of the adrenals, which produces excessive quantities of certain hormones affecting the blood pressure.

A very rare adrenal gland tumour — *phaeochromocytoma* — secretes large quantities of the stress hormones adrenaline and noradrenaline into the bloodstream, producing sudden attacks of very high blood pressure.

(3) *Narrowing (coarctation)* of a section of the aorta shortly after it leaves the heart (see above) produces high blood pressure in the head and arms, and low pressure in the rest of the body. Present at birth, this condition is commoner in males and generally produces symptoms such as headaches, nosebleeds and aching legs between the ages of 15 and 30. The only treatment is an operation to remove the narrowed section of the artery.

(4) *Toxaemia of pregnancy* is a cause of hypertension in expectant mothers. A slight blood pressure rise during pregnancy is common, but antenatal check-ups always include measuring the blood pressure, in order to make sure that it does not exceed 140/90 mm mercury. Should this occur, the patient's progress is carefully monitored for early signs of toxaemia. These include fluid retention, first seen as severe ankle swelling and excessive weight gain; and protein in the urine. Specimens are tested routinely throughout pregnancy for signs of this, and also for glucose, blood or other abnormal constituents.

If signs of toxaemia appear, the patient is watched carefully, and advised to restrict her salt intake, and to rest and remain as quiet as possible. Hospital admission is essential if the condition worsens, because *eclampsia* — a form of epilepsy — can occur at an advanced stage of pregnancy and threaten the life of both mother and child.

Women who suffer from toxaemia of pregnancy stand an increased risk of developing hypertension later in life.

(5) *An excessive number of red blood cells* increases the viscosity (thickness) of the blood, and thereby the resistance to its flow and the pressure of the blood. The normal number of red cells is around five million per ml (millilitre) of blood, and a figure above six million is considered abnormal and termed *polycythaemia*.

Loss of plasma from the blood such as occurs in burn injuries increases the red blood count, because although the actual number of red cells is unaltered, the volume of plasma in which they are suspended is reduced. Their number also rises in response to oxygen shortage; this happens to people living at very high altitudes where the atmosphere is rarefied, and in others who suffer from severe heart and lung disease which prevents sufficient oxygen reaching the tissues.

In a rare condition known as *polycythaemia rubra vera*, the number of red cells can rise to nine or ten million for no accountable reason. Either some have to be drawn off, or the development of new red cells has to be prevented by means of drugs or radiation.

(6) *Certain drugs* can cause or worsen hypertension, including the contraceptive pill, steroids and non-steroidal anti-inflammatory drugs — NSAIDs — used to treat arthritis. The NSAIDs can cause fluid retention and a consequent rise in blood pressure.

Hypertension for which no cause can be found is called *essential* — a mild to moderately raised blood pressure is often symptomless, and only discovered by chance during a routine health check or insurance examination. A mildly raised blood pressure is not necessarily harmful in itself, but it can become more serious, and represent a serious threat to life expectancy.

Screening for hypertension

Clinically significant hypertension carries the same degree of risk as a raised blood fat (cholesterol) level, and experts in hypertension management recommend screening to detect asymptomatic patients.

About two-thirds of adults consult their doctor at least once a year, and over 90 per cent are seen at least once every five years. Routine blood pressure measurements, carried out at consultation if no recording has been made during the past five years, are now recommended in men and women aged 30 to 70 years.

There is no need to postpone having your blood pressure measured, though, until you next have something wrong with you! Often it is unnecessary to see the doctor: practice nurses carry out many routine blood pressure checks nowadays, and the earlier a high value is detected, the better, particularly if you are aged 45 or over.

A systolic blood pressure above 160 mm mercury, or a diastolic pressure above 95 mm mercury, increases the risk of developing coronary heart disease by a factor of five, compared with someone of the same age and sex but with normal blood pressure.

Risk factors

Blood pressure values fluctuate constantly. Stress is probably the commonest cause, and it is well-known that worrying that your blood pressure may be raised — a form of anxiety that reaches a crescendo as the sphygmomanometer cuff is wrapped around your arm — can rocket a normal blood pressure into the hypertensive range for the few important minutes involved in its measurement.

Few doctors prescribe antihypertensive drugs until a patient's blood pressure has been tested on three or four separate occasions. Patients who have rushed to the surgery for fear of being late are often asked to rest for 20 minutes to allow their blood pressure to subside. Orthodox blood pressure treatment is generally regarded as lifelong, and doctors prefer to be very certain that medication is necessary before starting therapy.

One theory about essential hypertension is that it results, in the early stages, from overstimulation of the sympathetic nerves (part of the autonomic nervous system) by prolonged exposure to stress and other factors. The resultant arteriolar wall spasm eventually causes structural changes that prevent these vessels from dilating in the normal way.

Certain factors, detailed below, are known to increase greatly the risk of essential hypertension developing.

Age

Blood pressure tends to rise as we grow older, the rate varying at different phases of our lifespan. There is a normal and fairly rapid increase from the low values of infancy to the higher values of childhood, adolescence and early adulthood, and graphs of the population's *average* blood pressure show a gradual, upward trend between the ages of 20 and 45 in both men and women, followed by a more rapid rise of 0.5 to 1.0 mm Hg systolic pressure per year until the age of 70.

It is possible, however, that the *normal* blood pressure increase between the early twenties and old age may be considerably less than is suggested by these findings. The majority of people develop some type of blood vessel disorder as a result of their diet, lifestyle or vulnerability to other risk factors, a fact to which their rising blood pressure gives testimony. The minority of people whose blood vessels remain disease-free throughout life show little sign of a rise in blood pressure as they age.

To claim that a person's blood pressure can be expected to rise from the age of 20 onwards is to claim that he or she can be expected to develop some degree of circulatory disorder or other kind of disease. Fortunately, even our risk-ridden, Western life style has not yet equated any type of illness — even those commonly affecting the majority of people — with normality.

Sex

Before you panic, this does not refer to sexual activity, but to gender! Hypertension in men is always more serious than in women, since their overall risk of developing heart or circulatory disease is greater. Referring to population averages, women have slightly lower blood pressure than men during their twenties and thirties, and slightly higher thereafter.

Possible reasons for this include hormonal changes, pregnancy, the use of steroid drugs such as the contraceptive pill and HRT (hormone replacement therapy) for menopausal symptoms, and perhaps a greater susceptibility to certain risk factors, such as weight increase, smoking, stress, and alcohol intake.

Race and environment

We are primarily concerned here with blood pressure problems in Western society. However, although most populations show an average age increase and distribution of pressure values similar to our own, certain racial variations provide an interesting comparison.

Most population studies carried out in East and West Africa, the USA, and the West Indies show similar proportions of hypertensive sufferers among black and white people, but some of the study samples indicate a considerably higher percentage among blacks. This contrasts with the results of studies carried out on the Indian subcontinent, where the number of hypertensive people is relatively low.

In some communities, the average blood pressure shows minimal tendency to rise with age — and the increase in blood pressure that does occur lacks the 'upward skew' of higher values found in Caucasians (see Fig. 2, page 30). Examples include East African nomads, South West African bushmen, and certain Pacific islanders such as the inhabitants of Pukapuka in the Northern Cook Islands. It is possible that diet, exercise, and an absence of the type of stress found in more developed societies provide a large part of the answer.

Obesity

Many studies have shown that putting on weight is associated with a significant rise in systolic and diastolic blood pressure, especially in young and middle-aged adults. Part of the reason is that, like every other body tissue, fat requires an adequate blood supply, and every pound of surplus fat increases the total length of the small blood vessels by approximately one mile! The heart is highly adaptable to many bodily changes, but the extra demands made upon it by a stone or more of excess fat are considerable.

Fortunately, loss of excess weight can reduce both high blood pressure in people suffering from hypertension and the chances of it developing in overweight people with a normal blood pressure. We will be looking at the safest and most reliable methods of weight reduction in Chapter 5.

Salt intake

The relationship between salt intake and hyptertension is uncertain. Severe hypertension tends to improve in response to a salt-restricted diet, while moderate to mild hypertension is inclined to worsen!

The suggestion that people with a family history of high blood pressure are especially susceptible in their blood pressure response to dietary sodium has been challenged by a number of research studies which have found no evidence of a genetic link. Some people do seem, however, to have an increased sensitivity to sodium, and further research is required to distinguish the nature of the link and to identify individuals most likely to be affected by a high salt intake.

CHAPTER 3

Hypertension and health problems

Hypertension is unusual, in that it is not an 'illness' in the usual sense, but a condition predisposing to the development of several disorders, some life-threatening. In addition, its early stages produce no symptoms; it rarely has an obvious cause; it can be controlled but seldom cured; it requires lifetime management; and the treatment itself may add symptoms.

One of the reasons that some doctors refrain from treating patients with mildly raised blood pressure is their reluctance to produce symptoms (i.e. drug side-effects) where none previously existed! Since all high blood pressure needs careful observation and control, the argument in favour of natural blood pressure reduction is particularly cogent.

It is essential to understand the risks hypertension imposes if you are going to make lifestyle changes to maintain or reduce its level. The younger you are, the greater the significance of a small blood pressure rise. If you are 35 and have a diastolic blood pressure of 100 mm Hg, your life expectancy is potentially reduced by 16½ years. If you are 55, this same blood pressure predicts 'only' a six-year reduction in life expectancy.

Some doctors prescribe medication for hypertensive patients of all ages. Other treat only those below 65, because of the problems inherent in the use of certain drugs (see Chapter 1) and because some research studies suggest that elderly patients are unlikely to gain any real benefit.

Fortunately, natural methods to reduce and control blood pressure can be used by people of all ages. A reduction in life expectancy of six years for someone aged 65 *may* seem small to medical statisticians, but it can seem very great when you reach that age and hope to enjoy years of healthy, active retirement.

Hypertension and ill-health

The disorders connected with hypertension are of two types. The first are largely the consequence of longstanding, abnormally high pressure inside the arteries, and include heart failure, kidney failure, and strokes. The second are caused by the arterial disease atherosclerosis, the development of which is greatly accelereated by high blood pressure; they comprise coronary heart disease and peripheral vascular disorders.

Coronary heart disease refers to the ill-effects upon the heart of diseased coronary arteries. Peripheral vascular disorders affect the 'peripheral' blood vessels some distance from the heart, such as the femoral arteries and their A- and B-road subdivisions supplying the lower limbs.

Heart failure

A moderately to severely raised blood pressure greatly increases the work-load of the left side of the heart, which endeavours to pump as much blood as usual into the aorta and the rest of the arterial system against the increased resistance offered by the constricted arterioles.

Muscles — including those of the heart — grow bulkier when used to excess, and one of the earliest signs of heart strain is a thickening of the wall of the left ventricle, the lower, left-sided pumping compartment from which the aorta arises. Enlargement of the heart can be detected by a physical examination, by a chest X-ray, and by an ECG (electrocardiogram), an electrical tracing of the heart providing information about its size and performance.

Eventually the effort proves too much, and the left side of the heart shows signs of failure. The blood supply to the organs and tissues is decreased, causing weakness and lethargy. The build-up of pressure in the left ventricle prevents the blood from the lung veins from flowing freely into the upper compartment (atrium), which drains into it, rather like a heavy traffic flow getting held up in its passage from one main road to another already overburdened by rush-hour motorists. The lung tissue becomes congested, producing a cough and breathlessness.

The cough can be dry or produce frothy, blood-stained phlegm — especially at night when attacks of acute choking and gasping get patients out of bed and leaning out of the window, terrified that they cannot breathe. The breathlessness is first noticed during prolonged exercise. Later, it accompanies mild activity and, when heart failure is severe, patients become breathless at rest.

Unless the raised blood pressure is reduced, and the left-sided heart failure relieved, the right side of the heart becomes affected. Pressure builds up in the right atrium, creating back pressure in the veins draining into it. A characteristic sign of this is enlargement of the external jugular veins on either side of the neck, returning blood to the heart from the scalp and face.

Their superficial position below the skin of the throat, where they offer such a convenient target for vampire attack in horror films, also makes them especially vulnerable to injury. They are partly visible in healthy people en route to the heart, starting just below the angle of the jaw, crossing large neck muscles, passing on either side of the Adam's apple (larynx) and finally disappearing into the chest behind the collar bone. Swollen jugular veins congested by backflow pressure show characteristic signs which help doctors assess the severity of heart failure.

Other signs of right-sided heart failure, all consequences of a congested blood flow, include swollen feet and ankles, an enlarged liver, loss of appetite, a swollen tummy, and passing less urine than usual.

Kidney failure

The relationship between kidney disease and high blood pressure is a classic vicious circle. Kidney disorders, especially those which interfere with their blood supply, can cause hypertension. Conversely, persistently high blood pressure (particularly the malignant type: see Chapter 4) can injure the kidneys. It damages their arterioles and impairs their function, which is highly dependent upon an adequate blood supply.

Large amounts of protein are found in the urine in hypertensive kidney failure. Symptoms may include getting up at night to pass urine, and passing larger than usual volumes during the day. In kidney failure, toxic substances usually filtered off and excreted in the urine collect in the bloodstream. The patient's condition can deteriorate rapidly and death can soon result. Unfortunately, treating the underlying hypertension rarely improves kidney function.

Strokes

A stroke consists of damage to an area of brain tissue as a result of pressure from escaped blood or interference with the circulation and a consequent shortage of oxygen and glucose. Brain cells depend for survival upon a constant and adequate supply of these two factors, neither of which they are able to store, and significant depletion severely injures the affected area.

Hypertension increases the risk of a stroke in two ways. First it encourages the development of *atherosclerosis* (see below), thereby narrowing the arteries of the brain. This heightens their chances of becoming blocked by a blood clot from the heart or lungs, or by a flake of tissue arising in the heart or a diseased artery.

Secondly, it places severe strain upon the walls of the brain's delicate blood vessels, and can eventually rupture one of them. If it does, blood escapes into the surrounding tissues, constituting a cerebral haemorrhage.

Symptoms of minor strokes include loss of use of a hand, arm or leg, and/or loss of speech. A more or less complete recovery is usually made within a fortnight, but lowering the blood pressure is mandatory.

Symptoms of major strokes include weakness or paralysis down one side of the body, speech loss, and sometimes loss of consciousness. The speech problems and paralysis persist for longer in a major stroke, but with help many people make a satisfactory recovery. Again, treating hypertension is a major priority.

Transient ischaemic attacks are similar to minor strokes and produce body tingles and numbness, speech difficulties, loss of awareness of identity and surroundings, lightheadedness, and visual disturbances. They can be very frightening, but the symptoms are over within a few minutes. They are thought to result from temporary spasm of the blood vessels supplying an area of brain, or from pressure upon an artery in the neck carrying the brain's blood supply, as a result of getting the neck into an unsuitable position.

One third of people who experience a transient ischaemic attack have no further trouble; a third continue to experience them from time to time without suffering severe consequences; and a third eventually have a more serious stroke.

Senile dementia is the fourth leading cause of death in Britain, and it affects between 5 and 7 per cent of the population over the age of 65 and 20 per cent of those aged 80 or over. It impairs physical movement and thought processes, memory, energy, emotional stability, appetite, and the ability and will to perform simple tasks such as dressing, preparing food or drink, and reading or knitting.

There are several different varieties of this disease, the one most pertinent to a discussion of hypertension being *multi-infarct dementia*. A series of minor strokes, which escapes the notice of the patient and his or her relatives and doctor, gradually destroys areas of brain tissue. Hypertension strongly predisposes elderly people to this condition, and argues in favour of reducing raised blood pressure within this age group.

Atherosclerosis

The development of fatty lumps, or plaques, in the walls of arteries impedes the passage of blood within. This process largely accounts for the vast problems of coronary heart and peripheral vascular disease, and its course and causes have been researched intensively ever since its connection with heart disease became apparent.

Despite this, understanding of the highly complex process of atherosclerosis is as yet incomplete. It is not a single condition, but follows different sequences in different arteries. Fatty streaks appear in the lining of blood vessels soon after birth. During the first ten years of life, the lining thickens, and small cushions of fatty material develop at points where the arteries branch.

These soft, yellow lumps reach maximal size and number between the ages of 20 and 30. One theory holds that they develop from a collection of monocytes — a type of white blood cell — which infiltrate the arterial lining, then engulf fat particles and other cells in their vicinity.

This sets the scene for the appearance of fibrous plaques, the hub of the atherosclerotic problem. Plaques start to appear in the arteries of susceptible people after the age of 20 and multiply as time passes, especially in high risk areas such as the coronary arteries and the cerebral arteries in the brain. They develop in the main from fatty streaks, a process which is sparked off, many experts believe, by some sort of damage to the arterial lining.

Blood flow turbulence is thought to cause this injury. Blood is pumped through the arteries at a rate of 1¼ gallons (5 litres) every minute, under considerable pressure. Some damage — especially in key areas such as arterial junctions where turbulence is high — seems to be inevitable. High blood pressure appears to be the most important factor aggravating the initial damage to the delicate vessel lining.

Platelets — small particles present in blood — clump together on the fatty streak or another damaged area, with the object of repairing it. They release chemicals which turn a protein in the blood, fibrinogen, into solid, hair-like threads of fibrin. These carry the repair task a step further by entangling white and red blood cells within their meshes, like fish in a net.

The result is a clot. Under normal conditions this process is counteracted, when it has gone far enough, by a powerful substance called *prostacyclin* produced by the arteries. This can be seen as a defence mechanism with which the arteries are equipped to prevent the formation within them of a dangerously large clot or thrombus. Sometimes, however, the platelets' repair facility becomes excessive. It overpowers the action of the prostacyclin, and a large thrombus is formed.

If high blood pressure continues to injure the arterial lining, a plaque develops, containing fibrous clot material and fats absorbed from the blood. This process illustrates clearly how many of the high risk factors co-ordinate to produce plaque disease.

While hypertension damages the arterial lining, high stress levels — themselves a major cause of hypertensive disease — release the hormones adrenaline and noradrenaline from the adrenal glands. High blood levels of these two chemicals in turn increase the blood's clotting tendency.

The human artery

In this context, the human artery itself is a hindrance rather than a help. It has been referred to as 'the worst made of all the mammals'. A vital aspect of atherosclerosis is the poor perfusion of the arteries' smooth muscular wall by oxygen and nutrients. Deposition of a fibrous plaque on its inner wall further reduces its oxygen and nutrient supply.

The transport of molecules through the arterial wall is another important factor. Human arteries often have patches where permeability to these molecules is particularly high. This problem, intensified by hypertension and the ageing process, weakens the arteries' ability to combat thrombosis.

Atherosclerosis is linked in many ways with diet — a factor that will be discussed at length in Chapter 5. A point of relevance to atheromatous plaque development, though, should be mentioned here. The process may be made worse by an immunological reaction to foreign proteins. Dr David Davies, a pathologist at the West Wales General Hospital, Carmarthen, oulined a long-term study in the newspaper *Doctor* (13 October 1983). He pointed out that death from myocardial infarction (heart attack) was sometimes associated with the presence of antibodies to milk in the blood of the victims. Male patients were found to have a threefold chance of dying from a second or subsequent heart attack if milk antibodies were present at the time when the first one occurred. The mechanism was not clear, but simple experiments had shown that milk proteins can cause blood platelets to clump together as they do during the initial stage of clot formation.

At the time of this report, Dr Patrick Gallagher from Southampton General Hospital had shown in laboratory experiments that the ability to tolerate soya protein reduced the incidence of atheroma threefold, although he was unable to support Dr Davies' milk antibody findings.

London GP Dr Jeffry Segall suggested that lactose (i.e. milk sugar) may cause coronary heart disease. He pointed out the relatively high number of people (83–98 per cent) in North West Europe capable of absorbing this substance, compared with the figure in Japan (22 per cent) and in other regions where the incidence of deaths from coronary artery disease is low.

Coronary heart disease

The heart never ceases its work of pumping oxygenated blood into the arterial system. Its muscular walls get a few moments respite during the diastolic (i.e. relaxation) phase between beats. Yet it contracts between 70 and 80 times per minute, day and night, for an average of 70 years and, in a few people, for as long as 100 years.

The walls of the heart consists of highly specialized muscular tissue with great durability and considerable strength, and in need of a constant and adequate oxygen supply. Other muscles are allowed to recover after exercise. If we are unfit and sprint a couple of hundred yards to catch a train or bus, the heart and lungs are unable to meet the sudden demand for extra oxygen-rich blood.

Our leg muscles are depleted of oxygen by the uncustomary activity and become painful, both on this account and because of the accumulation of waste products of metabolism (cellular activity). We are at liberty to rest them, though, until their supply of arterial blood is restored, the toxic chemicals are removed and the oxygen debt is repaid.

Unlike the calf muscles, the heart cannot rest after extra effort. It is, in fact, the source of its own blood supply! The coronary arteries bringing blood to its walls arise from the aorta, just as this vessel leaves the left side of the heart. The heart has to continue to pump in order for blood to flow along them and perfuse every area of its tissues. Coronary arteries narrowed by atheromatous plaques seriously limit cardiac (i.e. heart) function.

Angina

The chest pain that results from shortage of oxygen to the heart is a symptom about which a doctor should be consulted without delay. The pain can be intense, and may extend from the centre of the chest down one arm (generally the left) and up into the root of the neck. It can be triggered by sudden physical exertion, excitement, shock, or emotional stress, and is an advance warning of a possible heart attack.

Unstable angina is angina arising when you are at rest, or with increasing frequency and severity. Once thought to be caused by coronary artery spasm, intermittently disturbing their blood flow, it is now thought possibly to result from recurrent thrombosis in the region of a damaged fibrous coronary artery plaque.

In 1986, a Glasgow research team's paper in the *British Heart Journal* reported that squash players frequently continued with their sport despite being fully aware, having suffered attacks of angina, that the condition of their heart was inadequate to the demand. They had investigated 60 sudden deaths in the UK between 1976 and 1984, associated with squash. The victim's average age was 46 years, and ranged from 22 to 66. All were white, all but one were male, and the majority came from professional or executive families. Coronary artery disease accounted for 58 of the 60 deaths. All had many risk factors *the commonest of which was hypertension*. Overall, 45 of the victims had reported signs of heart disease, nearly always angina.

Heart attacks resulting from coronary artery disease are the commonest cause of fatality in many strenuous sports. Deaths occurring during marathon running, soccer, rugby football, basketball, and tennis have all been investigated. In one survey, they were responsible for 73 per cent of 109 deaths. Almost half of these occurred in men with well-documented risk factors, and one third had suffered from warning signs — known as 'prodromal symptoms' — such as extreme fatigue or anginal chest pain.

Experts urge all sports participants to seek medical attention for any untoward health problems, and evidence of damaged coronary arteries or impaired heart function means that they should stop playing that particular sport.

Heart attacks

Heart attacks end or cripple the lives of sportsmen and many others with coronary heart disorder. Known medically as *myocardial infarction*, or simply 'MI', they are caused in nearly all cases by severe narrowing of a major coronary artery by atheromatous plaques, and the eventual obstruction of that artery by a tear in its lining or by a clot (i.e. coronary thrombosis). The area of heart muscle (myocardium) deprived of blood becomes 'infarcted'; that is, it suffers irreversible damage due to oxygen and nutrient deprivation.

The extent of the myocardial infarct determines the severity of the heart attack: although massive ones usually kill, recovery following many is quite satisfactory, the damaged heart muscle undergoing repair by the formation of scar tissue.

Hypertension and a high blood fat (cholesterol) level are the two most important risk factors predisposing to atherosclerosis and heart attacks. Heart disease mortality figures are higher in the

UK than anywhere else in the world, the worst 'death spots' being Wales, Scotland, and Northern Ireland. Heart and circulatory disease kills more people in Britain than any other disorder, including all types of cancer grouped together, and claims one life every three minutes, i.e. 200,000 annually.

Changes in habit and attitude, a healthy diet, and a sound strategy for normalizing blood pressure can do much to improve this dismal outlook. They have already been put into practice on a large scale in the USA, Australia, New Zealand and Canada: countries with lifestyles similar to the UK and with comparable past records of heart disease mortality rates.

The heart attack death rate has fallen in some of these countries by up to 37 per cent. In the UK it fell by 3 per cent in 1986 compared to that of the previous year, but the overall figures for the past 15 years show a 3 per cent rise in the death rate among men *and a 10 per cent rise in the death rate among women*.

Before looking in detail at what can be done to improve the situation, we must place conventional medical treatment in its proper perspective. To do so, it is essential to understand its underlying rationale and the means by which antihypertensive drugs reduce and control high blood pressure, and this will be dealt with in the next chapter.

CHAPTER 4

The treatment controversy

Since hypertension was first known to predispose sufferers to heart attacks and strokes, several conflicting viewpoints about its treatment have struggled for supremacy. It is easy for uninformed people to dismiss this state of affairs by quoting cynically that 'doctors differ and patients die'. Nevertheless, controversy about medical treatment, although in many ways less than satisfactory, is in fact a healthy sign. It means that a great deal of research attention is being directed towards solving a certain problem — in this case, finding out all there is to know about hypertension and hypertensive patients, and establishing the most effective and safest treatment method.

Inevitably, when various theories are put forward and tested and new drugs are developed, the pool of knowledge assumes a murky appearance, with so many doctors and scientists earnestly stirring the waters, hoping the answer will soon reach the surface! The patients involved in surveys and clinical trials show varying group profiles; and, although computers analyse trial data, human beings rather than machines interpret them.

The further research progresses, the more experts are coming to realize the true complexity of hypertensive disease. Research into the problem has produced impressive results over the past 15 years, and although much remains to be done, it should not be too long before the answers to many important questions become clear.

According to experts — cardiologists, epidemiologists, physiologists, geneticists — speaking at the International Society of Hypertension (ISH) biennial meeting held in the summer of 1988, hypertension cannot be considered a single entity. It is now recognized as a final common pathway through which a number of complex and abnormal physiological processes — metabolic, genetic, environmental — manifest themselves. The fact that numerous possible causes exist explains why no single antihypertensive drug, or group of drugs, treats all sufferers satisfactorily. It also complicates treatment.

Mild and moderate hypertension

Mildly hypertensive people (i.e. those with a diastolic blood pressure between 95 and 105 mm Hg — see Chapter 2) were once considered better off without medication, at least initially. Speaking at an international symposium on hypertension in New Orleans in 1983, Professor Norman Kaplan from the University of Texas said that patients within this category had a low mortality, and that only three out of every thousand patients would benefit from medication. He pointed out that if drug therapy were withheld the blood pressure would fall spontaneously to below 90 mm Hg in about one-third of these patients.

Interestingly, he suggested lifestyle changes, including weight loss where appropriate, as the preferred approach, and drugs as a last resort only if the blood pressure remained above 100 mm Hg after six months.

Opinions remained divided on this issue for some time. The aim of treating hypertension is to reduce the incidence of angina, heart attacks, and other disorders discussed in the previous chapter. The rationale of treating mild to moderate degrees of hypertension did not start to become established until the early 1970s when a wide choice of antihypertensive drugs started to appear.

A series of long-term studies reported in the *Journal of the American Medical Association* in April 1988 produced scientific evidence of a valuable reduction in deaths in such patients from coronary heart disease as well as from strokes, heart failure, and kidney disease. A total of 3,234 male patients suffering from mild to moderate hypertension were treated in this research trial, know as the MAPHY study (primary prevention with metoprolol in patients with hypertension), either with a thiazide diuretic drug or with the beta blocker metoprolol (Betaloc, Lopressor).

They were followed up clinically for an average of 4.16 years; the reduction in blood pressure was equal in both treatment groups, but there were significantly fewer deaths from heart attacks and strokes among those patients given the beta blocker.

Women and hypertension

The treatment of women with high blood pressure is given special consideration in many reports. Some research trials have indicated that women with mild to moderate hypertension benefit less than men from drug therapy. In one study conducted by the British Medical Research Council which included 9,048 men and 8,306 women aged 35 to 64 years, the patients were treated with either a placebo (dummy), and diuretic, or a beta blocker drug, and were followed up for 5½ years.

The rate of strokes and cardiovascular problems fell significantly in both sexes, and response to drug treatment was similar in a number of ways. However, while the overall death rate was reduced among male patients by active treatment, it was increased among females (but see the Amery study mentioned below).

Reasons for the latter finding may include increases in the consumption of alcohol and in smoking by women. Both increase the risks of high blood pressure, and so does obesity. Women who drink more than the recommended amount (see Chapter 9) and/or quit smoking tend to put on more weight than men — one study showed an average gain of 21 lb (10 kg) in women who had abandoned cigarettes. This is a major deterrent to would-be non-smokers, and emphasizes the need for a healthy, calorie-controlled diet and exercise to combat overweight (see Chapter 5).

The elderly and hypertension

There is now substantial evidence that active treatment of mild to moderate hypertension in elderly people reduces the risks of associated ill-health and death. The Veterans Administration (VA) studies of 1967, 1970, and 1972, which were confined to males, suggested that the elderly derived the same benefits from blood pressure reductions as younger individuals.

The Australian study of mild to moderate hypertension (National Heart Foundation of Australia, 1981) backed this finding in their male participants, and the 1985 European study carried out by A. Amery and colleagues and reported in *The Lancet* showed unequivocally that treatment benefited elderly patients. It reduced cardiovascular deaths by 37 per cent in those with a diastolic pressure of 90–99 mm Hg, and by 50 per cent in those with a diastolic reading between 100–119 mm Hg *in both sexes*.

However, these benefits decline with advancing age, so that treating uncomplicated hypertension (i.e. hypertension that is not causing apparent harm), in the over-80s is probably unjustified. Specialists suggest the careful selection and monitoring of antihypertensive therapy in old people to ensure that the side-effects of medication do not impair the quality of life.

Choice of medication

Malignant hypertension

Malignant or 'accelerated' hypertension is a medical emergency requiring immediate treatment. The diastolic pressure is frequently in the range of 130 to 170 mm Hg, and the patient often feels very ill, common symptoms including headaches, giddy spells, blackouts, breathlessness, and blurred vision.

The retina of the eye is damaged and the optic nerve disc is swollen (papilloedema). This the physician detects by examining the retina through the pupil of the eye with a lighted instrument (ophthalmoscope) in a suitably darkened room.

There may be evidence of kidney or heart disease, and hypertensive encephalophy — generalized brain swelling due to leakage of blood plasma through the walls of damaged brain arterioles — is another serious complication.

Most patients with malignant hypertension are hospitalized at once. Gravely ill patients requiring immediate blood pressure reduction may receive an intravenous injection or drip infusion of labetolol (Trandate), a combined alpha and beta blocker (see below). The rate of administration is carefully monitored because it is dangerous to reduce the blood pressure too rapidly.

'Stepped care' treatment

The 'stepped care' method of treating all patients with mild to moderate hypertension emerged in the early 1970s, and provided

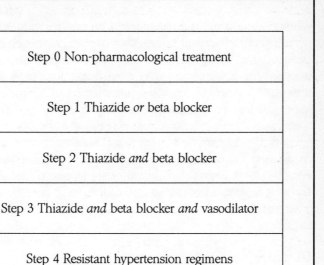

Step 0 Non-pharmacological treatment

Step 1 Thiazide *or* beta blocker

Step 2 Thiazide *and* beta blocker

Step 3 Thiazide *and* beta blocker *and* vasodilator

Step 4 Resistant hypertension regimens

Fig. 3 'Stepped care' treatment

doctors with a sequence of therapeutic manoeuvres which would ensure the reduction of blood pressure to a satisfactory level. Step 1 was generally a diuretic at less than full dose, step 2 was the diuretic at full dose and step 3 was the addition of methyldopa, reserpine, or a beta blocker. If control remained unsatisfactory, further drugs were added or substituted until the desirable blood pressure was achieved — see Fig. 3.

As W.A. Littler, Professor of Cardiovascular Medicine at the University of Birmingham, points out in *Cardiovascular Focus* 22, Bayer UK Ltd, the success of any regimen depends ultimately upon patients' compliance; 50 per cent of patients with symptoms and 60 per cent of patients without symptoms do not take the drugs as directed. The simpler the treatment, the more likely the patient will be to remain on therapy and take it as prescribed.

As new antihypertensive drugs were developed, the original stepped care schema underwent several changes, with vasodilator drugs such as hydralazine (Apresoline) replacing those at step 3. By the end of 1985, the massive amount of information that had been obtained from trials and studies on hypertensive treatment placed stepped care policy under careful scrutiny. Today's approach is far broader, and its most interesting aspect is step 0, which refers to natural blood pressure control methods.

Professor Littler (and many other experts) now feel that a more individualized approach to hypertensive patients should be adopted in preference to a 'slavish pursuit of a prescribed regimen'. He advocates *more non-pharmacological (i.e. natural) techniques for the management of mild hypertension*, and emphasizes that the patient's quality of life must always be borne in mind.

Clinical studies have shown that the more recently introduced drugs — alpha blockers, combined alpha-beta blockers, calcium antagonists, and ACE inhibitors — are as effective at controlling blood pressure as many of the older ones. Initially they were assigned to steps 3 and 4 in the stepped care programme, but experience with the calcium antagonists and ACE inhibitors suggests that they should be considered much earlier on: they can be used alone, together, or with diuretics or beta blockers, and are thought to have advantages over these last two traditional standbys.

Doses of all drugs are now kept as low as possible, and given in time-release form wherever possible. This allows a once daily dose to be taken.

Patients, doctors and medication

Few patients are told enough about the medication they are expected to take. Certainly no doctor can be expected to give each patient a mini-lecture in physiology and pharmacology; but at least people need to be told which drugs are being prescribed for their condition, what these drugs can be expected to do, and possible side-effects to watch out for.

Consultation time during busy surgeries does make this difficult; and some doctors understandably object to reeling off lists of side-effects to their patients, on the grounds that the power of suggestion alone can produce an impressive display of symptoms in anxious, stressed, highly imaginative people. The solution is, of course, to explain just what is necessary, avoiding over-lavish discussions of adverse reactions which, although described in the drug literature, are frequently very rare.

It is only when doctors co-operate with patients and treat them as intelligent human beings that compliance with medication regimens can be expected to improve. It is also the only sure way to convince hypertensive patients who feel perfectly fit of the necessity of following medical advice.

How antihypertensive drugs work

Here, then, is how the main groups of antihypertensive drugs go about reducing blood pressure. Skip this section if you prefer; but becoming more familiar with whatever medication you are presently taking may encourage you to take it as prescribed, and/or make you determined to set complementary self-help methods into operation from this moment onwards!

Most antihypertensive drugs work in highly complex ways. The following is a brief and highly simplified summary of how the most important ones reduce blood pressure.

Diuretics act on the kidney tubules and cause sodium and water excretion, thereby reducing the volumes of the blood plasma and the extracellular fluid bathing the tissue cells. Extra urine is passed, the peripheral resistance due to constricted arterioles is lowered, the strain on the heart is reduced, and the blood pressure falls. Low doses of diuretics work as well as high doses, and produce fewer side-effects.

Black people generally respond better to diuretics than to beta blockers as initial treatment for hypertension, and a diuretic is therefore usually chosen for treating them unless there are contra-indications to its use.

Beta blockers, properly called 'beta-adrenergic blocking agents', counteract the blood pressure raising effects of noradrenaline produced by the adrenal glands. They compete with this stress hormone for action upon highly specialized 'beta-adrenergic receptor cells' which play significant roles in the control of blood pressure. Highly responsive to noradrenaline, which increases blood pressure, these cells are widely distributed throughout the body, and are found in particularly large numbers in the heart, lungs, and blood vessels.

The explanation of precisely how these drugs lower blood pressure is poorly understood, but it is thought that the heart's output of blood (cardiac output) is reduced without the usual compensatory 'clamping down' of the arterioles. In addition, the kidneys release less renin and this also causes blood pressure to rise.

Although they lower the 'useful' type of blood cholesterol (the high-density variety) and are unsuitable for asthmatics and people with defects in the heart's electrical conducting system, beta blockers are currently preferred by many doctors for step 1 therapy in white people, especially in cases where diuretic drugs are inappropriate.

Vasodilators — since the main problem in hypertension is increased resistance to blood flow because of constricted arterioles, the use of drugs that directly dilate arterial vessels seems the most logical approach to treatment. (This is a point which illustrates the scientific approach of allopathic medicine. Holistic — i.e. alternative — practitioners would strongly disagree, pointing out that tight-walled arterioles are in fact a *symptom* of a deeper, more complex problem affecting the entire person. However, here we are considering how orthodox medicines work and the reasoning — valid according to its own underlying premises — of how the particular illness in question arises.)

Vasodilator drugs have a relaxing effect upon the smooth muscle of the arteriolar walls. This lessens peripheral resistance and lowers the blood pressure. Hydralazine (Apresoline) becomes tighly bound to the blood vessel walls and acts for longer than some of the others. Vasodilator therapy is used in combination with a beta blocker and diuretic to treat moderate to severe hypertension.

Calcium antagonists, like vasodilators, lower resistance and blood pressure by relaxing constricted arterioles. Their action relies upon inhibiting the passage of calcium ions (electrically charged calcium atoms) into the smooth muscle walls.

They can be used alone (see above); or nifedipine (Adalat) and nicardipine (Cardene) may be prescribed together with beta blockers. They are useful for patients suffering from diseased arteries of the lower limbs; and for asthmatics, for whom beta blockers are generally unsuitable.

ACE inhibitors work by combating the action of the enzyme responsible for converting the relatively inactive substance angiotensin I into its more potent form, angiotensin II. The latter acts powerfully on the arteriolar walls, making them constricted and narrow, and raising the blood pressure. They also reduce the production of the hormone aldosterone by the adrenal glands, resulting in extra sodium and water being excreted by the kidneys (i.e. a diuresis).

ACE inhibitors lower both diastolic and systolic pressure in all grades of hypertension, maintain the blood flow in the blood vessels of both brain and heart, and rarely cause postural hypotension. Unlike beta blockers, they are safe for both asthmatics and diabetics. They do not affect cholesterol blood levels, and neither deplete the body's potassium stores nor predispose it to gout or to hyperglycaemia (raised blood sugar levels — the diabetes problem).

Patients taking ACE inhibitors seldom complain of adverse effects. They are effective in all grades of hypertension, including severe forms which have failed to respond to other forms of treatment.

Alpha blockers counteract the constrictive effects of noradrenaline upon the arterioles by competing for attachment to alpha-receptor cells in the walls of these vessels. They are especially useful for controlling hypertension associated with excessive amounts of adrenaline and noradrenaline in the blood.

Combined alpha and beta blockers control blood pressure by alpha effects and by concurrent beta effects (see above) upon the heart. The systolic blood pressure rise that normally accompanies exercise is reduced, although the diastolic rise remains the same as usual. Drugs of this type benefit hypertensive patients with co-existing angina, and are suitable for treating hypertension of all degrees of severity.

PART TWO:

Reducing your blood pressure naturally

CHAPTER 5

Diet and weight control

On 18 January 1986, the weekly GPs' newspaper *Pulse* published an article entitled: 'Hypertension: Which Drug For Which Patient?' by Dr Richard Pearson, consultant physician at St Bartholomew's Hospital, London. In it, he commented:

> Recently, there has been immense interest in the use of non-drug treatments as adjuncts *or alternatives* [my italics] to drug therapy. A wide range of interventions has been shown to reduce raised blood pressure, but not all have been shown to reduce its complications.
>
> Following this advice will often allow patients to be treated with smaller doses of drugs than they would otherwise need. This will lead to better tolerated treatment, better compliance and better control but it is unlikely to obviate the need for drugs in most cases.

The writer is being wisely cautious. Many patients with moderate to severe hypertension, especially when it has been long established (as well as a few with the mild variety), *do* require continuous medication. If this turns out to be true in your case, be cheered by the prospect of reducing the doses of drugs you are taking, and thereby any side-effects you may experience.

Remember, too, that hypertension is a highly complex condition, and that each hypertensive patient is an individual with his or her own built-in capacity to respond to natural therapy. It may seem unlikely, for a variety of reasons, that *you* will be able to stop medication altogether. But natural treatment frequently produces unexpected improvements, and will certainly increase your general health.

Regarding the effects of natural treatment on the complications of hypertension, this must depend upon the severity and duration of the problems involved. Successful blood pressure reduction relieves the strain on the heart, and a mild degree of failure is reversible. Serious damage to kidney, eye (see malignant hypertension in Chapter 4), or brain, is beyond the scope of most experts, orthodox or complementary, to reverse.

Dr Pearson goes on to comment upon the benefits of weight loss, exercise, relaxation, ceasing to smoke, and reducing alcohol intake, and states: 'Dietary modifications have been widely advised and are generally accepted.'

Diet: its aims

The word 'diet' has a doleful ring. Litanies are sung in the praise of every one invented, yet disillusion invariably sets in if they are regimentally organized and too demanding. Perhaps diets, as popularly interpreted, are the one health control method the majority of people are eager to try, and the one most often abandoned as unsuccessful and depressing.

'Dietary modifications' sounds even worse. This usually refers to a restricted eating pattern designed for weight reduction, or the control of diabetes or some other illness. The dictionary definition of diet, however, puts the matter into a welcome perspective. It is, simply, 'the usual food and drink of a person or animal'. So we will continue to use this convenient shorthand term for a way of eating that is 'modified' with four main aims in view. These are:

(1) to improve general health, increase vitality and boost energy
(2) to reduce high blood pressure
(3) to reduce a high serum cholesterol level
(4) to reduce and stabilize body weight.

While the first two will apply to you, the last two may not. We did see in the last chapter, though, that in Britain the *average* serum cholesterol tends to be way above that of other populations with a low incidence of heart disease; so there is every reason to keep a careful check on your own levels.

Similarly your weight may be ideal, or even on the low side, for your height and build (notice that I do not mention age — we will look at this in more detail in the final section). You are to be envied or congratulated, depending upon your metabolism or your self-control! Nearly 40 per cent of men and 33 per cent of women in the UK are overweight, according to the guidelines for body weight provided by the Royal College of Physicians' 1983 report *Obesity*.

You may eat normally and have no need to count calories. If you maintain your normal-to-low weight by stringent diets, however, you will be able to reject these time-wasters in favour of a healthier and more acceptable eating pattern that will control your weight naturally.

Whole foods and public attitude

Whole foods are the subject of as much controversy among the population at large as aspects of hypertensive treatment are among doctors!

Support for natural foods is growing. Over the past five years, consumption of full-cream dairy products, white bread, red meat, and eggs has fallen, and demand for wholemeal bread, low-fat sausages, skimmed milk and reduced-fat dairy products, and fresh fruit and vegetables has increased. This trend must partly account for the slight decline in the gradient of the heart attack death rate which, in 1986, had dropped by 3 per cent compared with 1985.

You may already be a whole food enthusiast. Some people, however, detest the term, relegating it to a minority of yuppie health cranks with plenty of time to follow weird recipes and ample cash to spend on ingredients.

'Anti whole fooders' see no point in altering their usual diet, and continue to relish their fish and chips, chocolate bars, commercial icecream, and sliced white bread. They maintain that no one in the family will eat wholemeal bread, and that it goes off quickly; that raw fruit takes too long to chew when a quick snack is needed; that the fresh vegetables need preparation and longer cooking time than their frozen or canned equivalents; and that life is not worth living without food you can look forward to and enjoy!

The inappropriate moral attitude that some whole food enthusiasts, in common with many non-smokers, have assumed is partly responsible for this reaction. Health zealots, among them certain food manufacturers who make 'additive absence' their selling point, dogmatize what is no more than a sane and practical way of eating.

Smug proselytizing is useless — and may endanger the nation's health! It reinforces people's determination to carry on as before. Assertive types condemn all health advice as rubbish, while the more timid, equally determined not to be dictated to, simply dive underground, taking their habits with them!

Sensitive smokers in small communities have been known to whisper a request for 20 of their favourite brand at supermarket checkouts, hoping no one in the queue behind will notice the transaction! This is how embarrassed young girls often behaved in the 1950s when buying a packet of 'STs' (sanitary towels)! At this rate, the courageous purchasers of sliced white bread will soon be burying their loaves at the bottom of their baskets, and smuggling them out via the fire exit!

Whole food eating is not a religion. It ordains neither priests nor preachers, and promises no health paradise for those who keep its commandments! But you'll follow its guidelines *if* you are convinced the results will be worthwhile. A whole food diet, together with other measures, will increase your energy and resistance to illness, and help to reduce your blood pressure. You may even find it brings an end to bimonthly prescriptions for antihypertensive drugs!

What are whole foods?

They are foods to which nothing has been added, and from which nothing has been removed. They are *the* foods for everyone who desires to remain or to become as healthy as possible. They are collectively the natural human diet, unimpoverished by efforts to improve their colour, flavour, texture, and durability. And they are superabundantly rich in the nutrients — vitamins, minerals, trace elements, fibre, and amino acids — essential to human biochemistry.

Research has produced a score of international reports recommending changes in our present way of eating, and emphasizing the dietary significance of whole foods. Two British Government reports, NACNE (the National Advisory Council on Nutrition Education) and COMA (Committee on the Medical Aspects of Food Policy) have agreed the findings. Futher studies have shown that whole foods guard against obesity, stomach and bowel disease, allergies, depression, chronic fatigue, certain cancers, diabetes, and many other disorders, and can help to relieve them once they have developed. They are highly beneficial to the circulatory system, and therefore to people suffering from high blood pressure.

Up to and including the first decades of this century, everyone ate whole foods because there was nothing else! Wholemeal bread; fresh meat, poultry, fish and eggs; milk, butter and cheese; vegetables and fruit were everyday fare, and the food with which our grandparents and great-grandparents were familiar throughout their lives.

Far from today's technology improving the flavour of real food, it is far more apt to destroy it. Elderly people today who remember a different era are correct when they claim that food today does not taste as it once did. Battery egg production, crop pesticide sprays, the hormone treatment of farm animals, and food processing techniques are among the many factors that impair the flavour, texture, and nutritional value of the modern diet.

Certainly malnutrition was a grave problem in past times for the underprivileged. Epidemics of infectious illness caused many more fatalities than they would today, and rickets (a bone disease caused by vitamin D deficiency) was rife among poor children during the Industrial Revolution.

Of greater relevance here, however, is the fact that heart disease was virtually unknown at the turn of the century. Canadian Baronet Sir William Osler, probably the most brilliant physician of his time (1849–1919), admitted that he would find the condition harder to diagnose than many others, since he had seen no more than a small handful of cases throughout the whole of his professional life.

Ironically, the problem of malnutrition is still with us. Much of what we eat is lacking in essential nutrients. We eat far more fat and sugar, about the same amount of protein, and far less natural carbohydrate. We eat fewer potatoes and less bread 'because they are fattening' (but see below), less fibre, and fewer grains, vegetables, and fruit.

Many aspects of our modern lifestyle can be held responsible for the present epidemic of coronary heart disease. Among them, our diet, especially with the ready availability of high fat and high sugar processed convenience foods, is considered by many health experts to be the chief culprit.

(1) Improved health and vitality diet

You may wonder where vitality comes into the picture! Perhaps you connect it with active, sporty youngsters keen on marathon runs, aerobics classes and all-night disco dancing! You can, and should, feel 'vital' at any age, and as full of energy and 'go' as your personal circumstances permit. Whether you are 40, fat and fed-up, or 70, stressed and sceptical about natural blood pressure control methods, vitality, well-being and zest for life are your birthright. This can return as if by magic with the appropriate diet, adequate relaxation, and effective blood pressure reduction.

Eating for health and vitality

The most important points of whole food eating are:

- the elimination of junk snacks and processed convenience foods from which fibre, vitamins and other nutrients have been removed, and to which synthetic chemicals have been added
- reduced intake of fat of all types, particularly the saturated animal type present in red meat and the skin of poultry; milk, butter, cheese, and other dairy products
- reduced intake of refined sugar
- reduced intake of salt
- more fibre.

Carbohydrates include sugars and starches, the latter being converted into sugar during digestion. The average Western diet favours the refined variety, i.e. white sugar which provides nothing beyond energy calories, and white flour which lacks fibre (some of the other nutrients removed during manufacture are replaced before it is sold!)

We are keen on white bread, rolls, baps and buns and other white flour products, e.g. pizza bases, pasta, shop-bought cakes, pastries, and biscuits. White rice is our favourite grain, and popular forms of potato include greasy chips and 'instant mash'. Sales are high of packet white sugar, pre-sweetened cereals, fruit canned in syrup, jams, marmalades, preserves, packet desserts, confectionary, ice cream, fizzy drinks, and alcohol.

Whole food carbohydrates are the complex, unrefined variety containing their full complement of fibre, minerals, and vitamins. Wholemeal flour is produced by milling the whole wheat grain including both the bran and the wheatgerm — the central 'life core' of the plant which contains essential fatty acids, vitamins B and E, calcium, and iron; and '81 per cent' wholemeal flour, used for making choux pastry, light sponges, etc, is the same thing with some of the bran removed.

Other unrefined carbohydrates include brown rice and other grains — buckwheat (strictly speaking, a seed), barley, oats, corn or maize, rye, wheat, millet; pulses — chickpeas, beans, peas; potatoes and root vegetables; and fruit — raw, dried and canned in juice. Nutritional experts now suggest that foods of this kind should make up 60 to 70 per cent of the total diet.

Foods high in simple sugars, such as sweets, chocolate, and canned drinks, raise the blood sugar level rapidly, especially when taken on an empty stomach. They raise the spirits, which is why they are chosen as comfort foods, and supply instant energy. The problem arises once the sugar has reached the bloodstream — a sudden rise in sugar causes the pancreas gland to release a burst of the hormone insulin. This drives the extra sugar out of the bood and into the tissue cells and, when the influx of sugar is sudden and very great, this can occur so efficiently that the level in the blood drops equally suddenly, often to an abnormally low level. A low blood sugar level (hypoglycaemia) brings on unpleasant symptoms such as a rapid heart beat, nausea, headache, plus the need for more sugar — quickly. This cycle may be repeated several times until the next full meal is eaten. Binge-eating sugary foods is thought to be one of the causes of non-insulin-dependent diabetes developing in middle age.

Whole food recipes are sweetened with chopped dried fruit, grated raw fruit, and fruit concentrates. Unrefined brown sugar, molasses (black treacle), honey, maple syrup, and carob powder (a natural chocolate powder substitute) are also sometimes added.

Fibre lends food consistency, making it chewy and filling. It absorbs water and swells, curbing the appetite; and it bulks out the bowel motions, guarding against constipation. Certain types line the stomach wall, reducing the absorption and digestion of cholesterol and other dietary fats. They also control the entry of sugar into the bloodstream, at a rate at which the pancreas can cope. The result is a constant supply of energy without hypoglycaemic symptoms.

The best sources are beans, lentils, whole grains, fresh fruit and vegetables, dried fruit, and wholewheat bread. Sprinkling bran on cereals or adding it to other foods is unsatisfactory, because its phytic acid content impairs calcium absorption and can lead to calcium deficiency.

In developed countries, fibre-deficient diets are the most important cause of chronic constipation, and the resultant accumulation of toxins in the large bowel has been associated with cancer in a number of studies. Too little fibre is also related to other forms of cancer, varicose veins, atheroma, and other circulatory problems. The recommended daily intake of fibre is 25–35 g.

Protein is needed by the body for numerous biochemical processes, including repair activities and the generation of new cells. It also supplies energy at the same rate as carbohydrate, 1 gram generating about 4 calories. Red meat, especially beef and lamb, figure extensively in our diet in the West and it is classified as a 'first class' protein source because it provides all the essential amino acids (protein building blocks) we require.

However, red meat is broken down during digestion into certain substances which are thought to be connected with disorders of the large bowel, and it supplies more saturated animal fat than it apparently contains. Besides the rind of fat around a steak or joint, the flesh of farm-reared animals is marbled throughout tis substances by layers of fat. Interestingly, this does not occur in the flesh of wild animals — rabbit, hare, venison, wild boar — living in their natural habitat. Predictably, the latter benefit from a natural diet and adequate exercise.

The healthiest sources of protein for non-vegetarians include poultry with the skin removed, game, kidneys, liver, heart, and fish. Oily fish such as mackerel, kippers, herring, sprats, salmon, whitebait, and sardines, are especially beneficial. The oil has been found to contain two rare essential fatty acids, one of which, EPA (eicosapentanoic acid) offers protection against arterial disease and heart attacks (see Chapter 6).

Eggs (three or four weekly), cooked without fat, low-fat cheese and soya products are also high in protein. Many meat-eaters eat plant protein for several meals a week from preference rather than for health reasons. They are delicious in hot and cold dishes, and pulses and grains are low in fat and rich in protein and fibre. they can be used with seeds, nuts, and dairy products (cheese, milk, yogurt) to provide all eight essential amino acids. (The soya bean is unique in containing them all.)

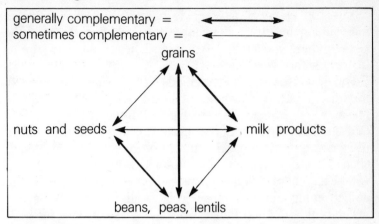

Sarah Brown, in her *Healthy Living Cookbook* (Guild Publishing, London), gives the above diagram to illustrate the complementary proteins.

The recommended daily intake of protein in the UK is 65-90 grams for men and 55-63 for women. Certain factors such as stress, infectious illnesses, excessive heat, and heavy physical labour increase our individual needs.

Fat delivers more than twice the number of calories produced by carbohydrate or protein — around 9 calories per gram. This is what makes fat a dieter's worst enemy. There is no recommended daily intake for fat in the UK in terms of grams/day, but some nutritional experts believe that a healthy adult between the ages of 20 and 50 should reduce his or her intake to below 10-15 per cent, in contrast to the average consumption in Britain of about 40 per cent per day.

A whole food diet that limits the intake of red meat and full-cream dairy products automatically reduces the intake of saturated fat. This, together with its high appetite-satisfying fibre and low refined sugar content, make whole food eating a natural choice for overweight people who want to shed surplus pounds, avoid hunger, and enjoy their food.

The healthiest sources of polyunsaturated fats (called PUFAs, or polyunsaturated fatty acids) are cold-pressed cooking oils such as safflower, sunflower seed, and soya bean oil, and margarine made from them — usually the soft, spreadable type. Cold-pressed plant oils have had more care taken in their preparation; high temperatures are used during the extraction of ordinary cooking oils, and these convert some of the beneficial essential fatty acids in the natural oils (known as *cis*) into useless *trans* forms. Cis essential fatty acids are used by the body in maintaining healthy cell membranes, including those of the tissues lining the arteries, veins and heart; the trans forms interfere with cis activities.

The healthiest cooking methods are those making use of minimal quantities of fat, and subjecting oils to hot temperatures for as short a time as possible. Stir-frying does require a tablespoonful of oil used, to be heated to a high temperature, but the whole procedure takes only a few minutes. Certain foods, such as kidneys, liver, oily fish, and some white fish, can be grilled with a coating of lemon juice instead of oil, without drying out; and steaming and boiling use no fat at all.

The health and nutritional benefits of these cooking methods can be best appreciated by contrasting them with, say, the three-hour roasting of a leg of pork, thickly surrounded and infiltrated with artery-clogging saturated fat; and with the alternating high and low temperatures to which a vat of fish and chip shop oil is subjected, at least for one opening period and maybe for weeks on end!

Drinks — beyond doubt the healthiest drink in the world is pure mineral water; probably the unhealthiest in the long run is alcohol (see Chapter 9). Between these lie the superbly nutritious vegetable and fruit juices you prepare and drink while fresh; and the canned and bottled fizzy rubbish, full of sugar or low calorie sweetener, often cola, and all manner of assorted dyes and artificial flavourings straight out of the manufacturer's chemistry lab! Shun them if you are health conscious.

Tea and coffee are ideally avoided, but this stricture is altogether too demanding and unrealistic. Tea may contain tannin and other noxious substances, but it remains the 'cup that cheers' and where would we be without the traditional cuppa? So, attempt to limit tea to three or four cups daily, preferably sugarless with a little skimmed milk.

Coffee lovers should remember caffeine in this beverage, and choose the healthier decaffeinated type — especially if you like your drink strong, and/or suffer from palpitations. Dandelion coffee suits some palates and is caffeine-free. Tisanes no longer taste of dry hay. Made from fruit, herbs, and flowers, they contain such exotica as wild cherries (full of vitamin C), hibiscus, rose buds, orange blossom, and passion flower leaves, and are as delicious as their beautifully decorated boxes suggest.

(2) Eating to reduce high blood pressure

Start eating whole foods and you are halfway towards a healthier heart and circulation. Here are some extra recommendations.

- Be extra vigilant about fat! Reduce the number of meals you eat that are based on meat, meat products, and dairy products, and remove all visible fat. Avoid frying and roasting, and remember the hidden fat in ready prepared foods, cakes, and biscuits.

- Include fish as often as possible. Try mackerel, herring, or sprats if you're unfamiliar with them as they are delicious grilled with a little mustard or vinegar. Shellfish are very healthy, although prawns, lobster, oysters, and scallops are expensive, so include the humbler shrimps, cockles, whelks, and mussels. Even winkles are not to be despised!

- Aim at eating a large salad of fresh raw fruit and vegetables daily. Avoid oily sauces and mayonnaise, and try lemon juice or cider vinegar, mixed with chopped fresh herbs and a little honey or low fat yogurt.

- Include natural sources of the mineral potassium — green leafy vegetables, tomatoes, potatoes, citrus fruit, bananas, honeydew melon, and sunflower seeds are good choices.

- Be extra vigilant about your calorie intake if you have a weight problem; avoid the empty calories clearly present in confectionery and 'hidden' in pies, cakes, and tarts. If you *do* yearn for chocolate, try a carob bar instead, available from health food shops and chemists. Substitute reduced-sugar jams, marmalades etc. for their full-sugar equivalents. Don't forget to include the calories they provide in your daily count.

- Eat less salt. Many of us eat around 12 grams daily, which is ten times more than we need. You can reduce your intake by ceasing to add it to food, and either getting used to the flavour or using a low sodium substitute. Many processed and tinned foods, cakes, cereals, biscuits, drinks, and desserts have added salt, so if you use these, check the label first.

- Reduce your consumption of alcohol (see how in Chapter 9).

- Don't forget your best friend, fibre! It's a good feeling to tuck into your breakfast porridge, homemade pea soup or savoury red kidney bean supper, knowing your food is helping to reduce your serum cholesterol level! Eat more baked potatoes, including the skin, and leave the peel on raw apples and pears (but wash them thoroughly). Try warm granary bread with a little low-fat soft cheese, and use pizza bases made of wholewheat flour. You won't have room for fattening sugary snacks between meals!

The whole secret of keeping to any eating plan is to pick things you enjoy. Make changes gradually, and introduce unfamiliar ingredients one at a time. Here are some ideas for meals to help you reduce a raised blood pressure.

On waking, a glass of fresh fruit juice or 'morning recipe' herbal tea. Then, for each meal, one of the suggestions listed.

Breakfast

Glass of fruit or vegetable juice/piece of fresh fruit.

Porridge with a little honey, molasses, fresh or dried fruit, or maple syrup.

Muesli with flaked wheat/millet/barley/rolled oats; fresh fruit/dried fruit, such as apricots, peaches, sultanas, raisins, currants; a few chopped unsalted nuts; seeds such as sunflower, sesame, pumpkin; skimmed milk; plain yogurt; mineral water or fruit juice to moisten.

Grilled kidneys/mushrooms/tomatoes or poached egg on wholewheat toast.

Piece of fish, steamed.

Whole grain bread/roll (wheat, barley, rye), with scraping of vegetable margarine/skimmed milk cheese; honey, low-sugar jam or marmalade.

Drink: water, fresh fruit juice, weak unsweetened tea or decaffeinated coffee.

Light meal

Large raw salad: use only fresh, attractive vegetables and fruit, avoiding any that look shop-weary. Mix green leafy vegetables (watercress, cress, lettuce in season, grated raw cabbage or Brussels sprouts, roughly shredded raw spinach) with any grated raw root vegetable other than potatoes, celery, fennel, raw mushrooms, beetroot, or courgettes. Dandelion leaves, celery, asparagus and parsley have a natural diuretic effect and are prescribed for hypertension by medical herbalists.

Add seeds as above (breakfast) or sprouts grown at home, and cold cooked grains or pulses, or wholegrain bread, as carbohydrate/fibre source. (Buckwheat is believed to help dilate constricted blood vessels and tone and repair vessel walls.) Raw fruit can be sliced in liberally, but go easy on bananas if you're trying to lose weight, and on avocado pears which are rich in oil.

Add a few unsalted nuts occasionally — cashews, peanuts, walnuts, Brazils — and chopped fresh herbs as often as possible. Non-oily salad dressings made with cider vinegar provide extra minerals and trace elements. Fresh garlic aids high blood pressure. For extra protein, a few shellfish, sardines, salmon or tuna drained of oil, or a little sliced turkey or chicken breast are good choices.

Drink: a glass of iced mineral water with a slice of fresh lemon or lime and some ice cubes complements raw food superbly.

Main meal

Whenever possible, start with a small raw salad as this may help small bowel digestion.

Vegetarian dish; braised liver or stuffed heart; small grilled steak (as a treat); fish, baked with herbs, grilled, cooked on plate over vegetables, as kegderee (any white fish, cooked and flaked), or cooked in foil with hot water, herbs, chopped garlic, slices of fresh lemon or orange and their juice. Curried egg; poultry, baked or casseroled (no skin).

Large baked potato with low-fat yogurt and herbs or skimmed milk cheese.

Large helping of lightly cooked vegetables, with pepper, lemon juice, a little vegetable margarine.

To follow: fresh fruit; fruit salad, fresh or canned in juice; custard made with skimmed milk and very little sugar; fruit crumble using wholewheat flour, a little natural brown sugar and pinch of nutmeg, cinnamon or ginger; homemade icecream made with low-fat milk; or slice of homemade cake.

Drink: mineral water, with ice and slice of citrus fruit; fresh fruit juice; 5 oz glass wine, or single measure of spirits with juice or low calorie mixer; or half a pint of beer or lager.

(3) Eating to lower a raised blood fat level

A raised blood level of cholesterol and/or triglyceride fats is termed hyperlipidaemia. Every laboratory has its own range of normal values but, generally speaking, normal blood cholesterol in adults is taken as between 3.6 and 7.3 mmol per litre (i.e. 140–280 mg/dl in the USA) and ideally between 4.5 and 5.2 mmol per litre (175–200 mg/dl). Normal blood triglyceride is 0.4 to 1.9 mmol per litre.

Four main types of the condition should be mentioned:

Primary hypertriglyceridaemia

This is an extremely rare disorder affecting children. They are unable to clear dietary fat at the normal rate, and chylomicrons (tiny fat particles) stay in the blood long after a normal meal. The blood triglyceride level is very high, but cholesterol levels are generally normal. Symptoms include bouts of pain after eating fatty food, an enlarged liver and spleen, and xanthomata (skin nodules).

Familial hypercholesterolaemia

This is the type of raised blood cholesterol running in families. It affects between 0.25 and 0.5 per cent of the population, and is associated with a greatly increased risk of coronary heart disease. Many patients suffer a heart attack before they are 30. Treatment generally requires both lifelong drug therapy, and dietary regulation.

Hyperlipidaemia of affluence

This is not a specific disease, but both very low density (VLDLs) and low density (LDLs) types of blood fats are raised. Most sufferers also tend to be overweight, and/or hypertensive.

There is insufficient evidence of the beneficial use of drugs for this condition, but some patients have been given the natural supplement guar gum to reduce their high blood fats. This fibre preparation is extremely viscous (thick and jelly-like) and is taken either in water with, or sprinkled on, every meal.

The main means of control is by diet. Many patients happily comply with dietary advice when the problem is explained to them, but many need help and persuasion!

Hyperlipidaemia secondary to disease

The blood cholesterol level is generally high in patients with the kidney condition *nephrotic syndrome*, and with an underactive thyroid gland. Treatment consists of relieving the underlying disorder. Raised blood fat levels commonly associated with overweight, gout, and diabetes are treated in the same way as the affluence condition.

The first three forms of raised blood fat level mentioned above are known as 'primary' because they do not occur as a result of a different underlying disease. The following dietary information is suitable for all of these.

Foods to be limited according to tolerance:

- lean meat, and poultry
- low-fat cheese, spreads e.g. *Gold*, and yogurts.

Foods to be avoided

- butter, margarine, cooking fats, and oils
- whole or semi-skimmed milk, egg yolks, cheese, icecream, cream
- cakes, pastries and biscuits made with fat
- sweets made with fat, e.g. fudge, chocolate, and lemon curd
- savoury snacks containing fat, e.g. crisps, peanuts, and olives and avocados
- offal, fatty and canned meat, meat products, fatty fish, and fish in batter, breadcrumbs or sauce

- soups, sauces, and products made with ingredients from this list.

Foods allowed freely:

foods not included in the above lists, e.g.

- skimmed milk

- bread and cereals

- fruit and vegetables and their juices

- natural fruit squashes and mineral water.

Table 1: Types of fat in commonly consumed foods	
Foods high in **saturated** fat	Foods high in **polyunsaturated** fat
butter, hydrogenated margarine, lard, suet, shortenings	sunflower, corn, safflower and soya oil
cakes, biscuits and pastries made with the above	foods made with above, omitting items in list opposite
fatty meats and meat products, offal	
whole milk, cream, icecream and chocolate	
crisps, most nuts, salad cream, mayonnaise	
full fat cheeses, egg yolks	

(4) Weight reduction

This is always a difficult problem, and no one is more aware of this fact than overweight people. If *you* are too fat, and have tried many times, unsuccessfully, to slim, your enthusiasm may receive the impetus it needs to succeed now that you realize the benefits to your health, life, and vitality.

Thousands of new diets are dreamed up yearly; many fall by the wayside, a few are sufficiently effective to become popular, and occasionally one such as the 'F-Plan' diet becomes firmly established in our repertoire of obesity treatment.

The secret of losing weight successfully is to pick the approach that suits *you*. Very low calorie diets (VLCDs) have been much maligned, but doubtless have an important role to play in certain cases. Most doctors feel they are better followed under medical guidance. Appetite suppressant drugs are rarely prescribed nowadays because of their side-effects, but used judiciously they can break the barrier of despair about weight loss failure, and set you on the path to steady weight loss.

Whatever means you employ, one single underlying equation is necessary for success. Calorie intake *must* fall short of energy output; and the wisest method is to combine regular exercise with a reduced-calorie diet.

Get a diet book that suggests the calorie intake appropriate to your sex, age, and degree of overweight. You may be surprised at the number of calories you are allowed to consume in the first few weeks. Very overweight men and women can normally lose weight initially on around 1,500 calories daily, depending upon how active they are. Clearly, an agricultural worker, building site labourer, refuse collector, or coalman expend more energy daily than a factory bench employee, shop assistant, or office worker.

As you lose weight, your metabolic rate (the speed at which your body burns food fuel) starts to fall and this can be remedied by regular exercise, if your lifestyle is generally inactive. Exercise is highly beneficial to weight loss, speeds the removal of surplus fat layers, tones heart and lungs, helps to reduce blood pressure, and — paradoxically — *increases* energy, alertness and vitality.

Follow either a normal whole food diet or one specially modified to reduce your blood fat levels to lose weight, reducing your calorie intake as extra pounds are shed.

In the next chapter, we will look at dietary supplements that help to reduce overweight and high blood pressure, and to lower stress.

CHAPTER 6

Helpful dietary supplements

For a long time controversies have raged, and they continue to rage, about the need for supplementing the diet with natural nutrients. Unexpectedly, the agonists and antagonists are not segregated exclusively on either side of the dividing line between orthodox medicine and natural therapists. Some nutritionally-trained medical experts support nutrient supplementation, and take the naturopathic view that even an exclusively whole food diet must frequently fail to supply every vitamin, mineral, trace element and amino acid that an individual requires.

A few alternative practitioners support so strongly the benefits of whole food eating that they discourage supplementation, and point those whom they advise in the direction of an increasingly assiduous search for a perfectly balanced eating regimen.

Doubtless, as is always the case, there are points of truth on both sides. Theoretically, a whole food diet, containing adequate daily amounts of fresh, organically grown fruit and vegetables, their freshly squeezed juices; seeds, nuts and pulses; free range poultry and eggs; and fresh fish from pure, uncontaminated river and sea water should supply every nutrient the human body requires.

Practically, though, such a diet is impossible to follow, simply because many of the foods are unavailable: concentrating one's imaginative faculties and intellectual powers almost entirely upon the wholesomeness of one's next meal can increase stress levels and produce neurotic obsessiveness, while the frustrated individual remains continually dogged in his or her attempts.

Malnutrition in the West

In addition to this problem, the Western lifestyle, though termed affluent, brings with it a unique type of malnutrition, even for those who attempt to eat healthily. Hidden salt, fat, and sugar are present in many proprietary brands of packet and frozen convenience health foods, and which of us, considering the pace at which most of us live, does not rely at least to some extent upon ready-prepared meals?

Stress plays a major part in all our lives from babyhood through to old age: the rising rate of stress-related diseases such as heart attacks, strokes and high blood pressure, psychosomatic illnesses, and neurotic and psychotic disorders bears witness to this. Animal and human research studies carried out over the past ten years in Europe, the United States, Russia, and Japan have shown that stress factors can have severely damaging effects upon both mind and body.

Once thought of as causing no more than tension and emotional problems, stress has now been shown to affect the function of the neurotransmitter brain chemicals carrying electrical impulse messages throughout the brain, the immune defence system, in particular the white lymphocyte cells responsible for combating infectious illnesses and malignant cell change, and the production of hormones, enzymes and other essential body chemicals. The sum total of the effects of stress greatly increases our need for many, if not all, vital nutrients.

Other disruptive factors — such as geopathic stress (magnetic earth meridians, ley lines, etc.); electromagnetic interference from overhead power cables, VDUs, microwaves, televisions and other domestic and industrial appliances; atmospheric pollutants; fatigue; tobacco smoke; chemically synthesized food additives; high alcohol consumption; radiation; and viral illnesses — also take their toll and increase our need for dietary supplementation.

Supplements for high blood pressure and the circulation

Whatever supplementation plan you follow, always start by taking one multi-vitamin/mineral complex daily. Specific dietary nutrients found to help reduce raised blood pressure, especially when taken in conjunction with a whole food diet and other health measures, include the following.

Vitamin E with selenium

Vitamin E has a number of beneficial effects throughout the body, particularly upon blood vessels. It acts as an anti blood clotting agent and as an antioxidant, counteracting the effects of free radicals (highly active molecule fragments) which injure and destroy many tissues throughout the body, and are thought to increase the rate at which fatty deposits of atheroma are laid down on the walls of arteries. This vitamin also promotes the production of normal red blood cells, and the healthy growth and development of every organ, including the heart and circulatory system.

Vitamin E combats hypertension by maintaining the health of the heart, arteries, veins and capillaries, and by encouraging the balanced control of the dilation and construction of the arterioles, largely responsible for the level of the diastolic blood pressure. Its actions in this capacity are reflected in its long established benefits to menopausal women suffering from hot flushes and night sweats. These symptoms, occurring under the influence of a falling oestrogen level, are believed to result from diminished control of the expansion and contraction of small blood vessels situated in and immediately below the skin. Vitamin E has no direct effect upon oestrogen deficiency, but acts as a regulator of abnormal blood vessel activity.

Vitamin E's actions in enhancing sexual and athletic performance, improving acne, and combating infertility are probably also related to its actions upon blood vessel function.

Natural sources include apricot oil, almonds, corn oil, cottonseed oil, hazelnuts (filberts), margarine, peanuts, sunflower seeds, wheatgerm, walnuts, and wholewheat flour.

How to take: doses of 100 IU daily, building up to a dose of 400 IU daily, over a period of eight weeks, have been used successfully to treat hypertension. Consult your doctor or a qualified nutritional expert if you are receiving medication of any kind.

Vitamin E supplements are often found in combination with the trace element selenium. Trace elements are vital minerals required by the body in minute amounts. Selenium complements vitamin E as an antioxidant, functions as an antioxidant itself, and also promotes normal growth and development. It is also speculated to offer protection against all ageing mechanisms, which must include the clogging of arteries with atheromatous deposits; and it helps to counteract cardiovascular disease, heart attacks, and strokes. It stimulates the immune defence system's cells, which also help to combat atheroma; it decreases platelet clumping in the bloodstream, and helps to prevent clot formation at the site of blood vessel damage in the heart and brain.

It occurs naturally in the following foods: wheatgerm and whole grain products, fish, liver and kidney, chicken, egg yolk, bran, broccoli, milk, mushrooms, cucumbers, garlic, cabbage, and onions.

How to take: No UK RDA (Recommended Daily Amount) has been established, but the quantities found in combination with vitamin E supplements have been calculated to supply normal daily requirements.

Carnitine

Carnitine is one of about 20 amino acid building blocks from which protein is made. Like other members of this group of compounds, it plays several important biochemical roles in human and animal biochemistry. The most important of these, in the present context, is the transportation of fatty acids into the power houses, (*mitochondria*), within which fatty acids and glucose combine with oxygen to produce energy.

According to recent research, carnitine appears to offer considerable benefit to the heart muscle of people suffering from atheromatous coronary arteries. Heart muscle cells are naturally rich in carnitine, one reason being that heart muscle derives between 48 and 70 per cent of its total energy requirements from long chain fatty acids. These energy requirements, even at rest, are considerable, for, unlike other bodily muscles, it can never take time off to relax. Over a 24-hour period, it pumps the equivalent of 1,800 gallons of blood through around 75,000 miles of blood vessels throughout the body.

High blood pressure strains the heart muscle, increasing its work-load and its energy requirements. In a recent clinical study, intravenous carnitine was administered to patients with ischaemic (coronary) heart disease. Their exercise tolerance improved, and their heart muscles were discovered to make more efficient use of fatty acids as energy fuel.

Carnitine can be taken as a dietary supplement for its protective effect against cardiovascular disease, and to help strengthen weakened heart muscle. A suitable dose for most adults, with the former aim in view, is 200 mg three times daily. Individuals suffering from heart disease or high blood pressure should obtain medical advice from a nutritionally-oriented medical practitioner.

Other amino acids

Histidine improves the flow of blood in the coronary arteries, and helps to lower an elevated blood pressure by relaxing blood vessel walls.

Taurine has been used successfully as a treatment for congestive heart failure, a common complication of longstanding hypertension, as explained earlier (pages 38–39). Over a four-week period, 58 sufferers took part in a controlled medical trial. Half of them received 'dummy' placebo tablets, while the rest received 6 grams of taurine daily. Those in the latter group experienced considerable relief from breathlessness, swelling and palpitations, while other benefits were noted in their chest X-ray pictures and in their overall functional capacity. Taurine proved useful whether or not the patients were receiving digitalis heart drugs. No significant improvement occurred in patients who received the 'dummies'.

In addition, taurine helps to keep cholesterol in solution in the bloodstream, rather than solidifying into plaques within arterial walls.

Fish oil supplements

These are known to contain *essential fatty acids* offering considerable and effective protection against heart and arterial disease. The most important is EPA (eicosapentaenoic acid), a continually high intake of which has been causally related to the low incidence of coronary thrombosis and other forms of heart disease in Greenland Eskimos, Japanese fishing communities, and other populations with a high consumption of oily fish.

EPA gives rise to compounds known as 3-series PGs, a class of prostaglandins, or hormone-like substances, which play vital roles in the minute-by-minute regulation of cellular processes throughout the body. The 3-series PG make blood clot formation (thrombosis) less likely, so EPA not only reduces the risk of heart attacks and strokes, but also lowers the levels of the class of blood fats and cholesterol most likely to give rise to fatty arterial plaques. It has also been shown to lower blood pressure, and to affect the activity of the monocytes (a class of white blood cell) which help to combat arterial disease throughout the body.

EPA may also help to reduce high blood pressure. One clinical trial involved 16 hypertensive patients over a 12-week period. All participants had a systolic blood pressure below 200 mm Hg, and a diastolic blood pressure between 91-100 mm Hg.

They were randomly allotted to one or other of two groups; all received a 'dummy' placebo oil, and a pure fish oil supplement in turn. The study was 'double-blind', i.e. neither doctors nor patients knew until the trial was over which patients had received olive oil placebo and which fish oil at any given moment during the study.

The average blood pressure of the patients, before they were allotted to their two groups, was 160/94 mm Hg. Following six weeks on placebo oil, this average had risen to 161/94.5 mm Hg; and after fish oil supplementation it had dropped to 151/92.5 mm Hg. In a reclining position, the systolic blood pressure was lower after fish oil extract than after olive oil placebo by an average of 5.48 per cent; and in a vertical position, i.e. standing, by an average of 5.66 per cent. The reduction in diastolic blood pressure following fish oil extract was not statistically significant.

Of the 16 patients, 13 found fish oil extract either as acceptable as, or more acceptable than, previous medication they had received for hypertension. The fish oil supplement used in this trial contained a higher concentration of EPA than those available in chemists and health food shops for a purely protective purpose; nevertheless, taking a daily fish oil supplement is a wise and healthy practice, whether your aim is to improve your overall heath, vitality, and cardiac stamina, or counteract high blood pressure naturally.

Evening primrose oil

Evening primrose oil contains the essential fatty acid GLA (Gammalinolenic acid) which also gives rise to helpful, heart-protective prostaglandins, this time of the 1-series (PGE1s).

Efamol is the brand that has been used in numerous clinical trials and studies evaluating the wide range of GLA's therapeutic applications, which have shown between 4 and 8 500 mg capsules of Efamol, taken daily, lower blood cholesterol levels, reduce the risks of thrombosis, and can be highly effective in lowering blood pressure in patients suffering from mild to moderate hypertension.

Coenzyme Q

This nutrient has attracted much research interest over the past decade. Coenzyme Q (CoQ) is an essential constituent of the cells' mitochondria, and it plays a vital role in energy production. Oxygen plays an essential part in the energy equation, and, as we have seen, unites with glucose and long chain essential fatty acids within heart muscular tissue, to release necessary energy. Specifically, it controls the flow of oxygen within individual cells, and therefore plays a major role in the metabolism of heart muscle.

Tests have shown that CoQ can lower blood pressure, relieve angina, and counteract congestive heart failure by enhancing the heart's muscular activity. Consult your doctor or a medically-qualified nutritionalist before taking this nutrient, if you suffer from heart disease or other circulatory problems.

Anti-stress supplements

Vitamin C with bioflavonoids

Vitamin C is the anti-stress vitamin par excellence. It boosts the immune defence system against the effects of physical, mental and emotional strain, and aids iron absorption essential to the production of haemoglobin, the oxygen carrying blood pigment, and of healthy red cells in the bone marrow.

It keeps the capillaries strong and healthy, and helps to guard against the weakness of their walls, leading to the leakage of blood following a bruise injury. Present in high concentration in citrus fruits, vitamin C was first discovered when oranges, lemons and limes were found to cure scurvy, the main symptoms of which are heavy bruising following minor injuries, and bleeding gums.

Other benefits of vitamin C supplementation include a reduction in blood cholesterol level, protection against heart disease, and improvement in emotional, stress-related disorders.

Natural sources of Vitamin C, besides citrus fruits, include: spinach, cabbage, broccoli, Brussels sprouts, watercress, green peppers (capsicum), kale, tomatoes, potatoes, paw-paws (papaya), guavas, rosehips, and blackcurrants.

How to take: Opinion varies enormously about the amount of vitamin C we should take as a daily supplement. Doctor Linus Pauling, the famous pioneer research scientist and Nobel prize winner, is reputed to have cured cancer with very high doses of intravenous vitamin C, and to take in the region of 21 grams daily himself. Generally, one gram daily, in addition to the vitamin C present in your multi-vitamin/mineral complex, should suffice; you should be able, safely, to double or treble this dose for a few days when symptoms of a cold, sore throat, or influenza appear, or when under heavy strain.

Bioflavonoids are the brightly coloured pigments in the skin and flesh of citrus fruits, peppers, apricots, cherries, grapes, paw-paws, tomatoes, and in green leafy vegetables. They are found in association with vitamin C, and include rutin, hesperidin, nobiletin, sinensetin, and tangeretin.

They, too, have an antioxidant effect, preventing the oxidation of vitamin C and adrenaline by copper-containing enzymes. They strengthen capillaries; prevent nosebleeds, post-partum (after birth) haemorrhage and easy bruising. They may also help to counteract retinal bleeding at the back of the eye in people with diabetes and hypertension.

How to take: No RDA has yet been established, but the amount present in vitamin C supplements is sufficient for normal purposes. Do not take it to rectify a bleeding problem with consulting your doctor first about the underlying cause.

Vitamin B complex

A need for B-complex vitamins increases generally when we are under stress. Supplementation with certain of them is known to offer particular value; unless advised differently by a qualified nutritionalist, you should take the entire complex in one supplement. Thiamine (vitamin B1) helps to combat emotional highs and lows. Niacin (vitamin B3) promotes the health of the entire nervous system, and helps to protect against both migraine headaches and stress-related high blood pressure. Pantothenic acid (vitamin B5) relieves tension, aids adrenal gland function, and combats anxiety and fatigue caused by subjection to physical/psychological stress. Pyridoxine (vitamin B6) can offer effective relief from tension and anxiety caused by the premenstrual syndrome (PMS).

Calcium

Many nutritional experts, doctors, and natural therapists recommend calcium supplements when stress levels are high, in order to meet the body's extra demands for calcium. Smokers and high protein eaters share an increased need for this mineral. Before, during and after the menopause, women are particularly in need of calcium, since a falling oestrogen level encourages bone thinning (oesteoporosis). The menopause, which generally occurs in the West around the age of 50, is also the age at which weight problems, cardiovascular disease, and hypertension are most likely to become apparent. The menopause itself also gives rise to additional tension, stress, worry and irritability.

Calcium supplements taken before retiring can help to ensure a sound night's sleep.

Magnesium

This has been dubbed the anti-stress mineral. It is essential for calcium and vitamin C metabolism, and should be taken with calcium in half the former mineral's dose.

The majority of people under stress require extra magnesium, while heavy drinkers need even more. Besides combating depression and tension, magnesium promotes the health of the cardiovascular system and helps to prevent heart attacks. (See *The Vitamin Bible*, Earl Mindell, Arlington Books 1985.)

Zinc

This mineral plays many essential roles in the body. It combats tension, helps to maintain mental alertness, and counteracts certain types of depression.

Weight reduction nutrients

Essential fatty acids

Evidence exists that certain essential fatty acids aid weight reduction by helping to turn dietary saturated (animal) fat into fuel, by increasing the rate at which it is consumed. A heavy carbohydrate consumption increases our need for this activity.

In particular, GLA (gammalinolenic acid), present in evening primrose oil (Efamol), has been shown to increase the metabolism of our brown fat layer. This type of body fat is found in various bodily areas, for instance on the upper back between the shoulder blades. The proportion of white fat to brown fat throughout the body helps to regulate the ease and the speed with which we lay down extra, unwanted fat layers. While white fat has a very low cellular metabolism, brown fat has a correspondingly high one. Increasing its fuel consumption capacity helps us to lose unwanted pounds and inches.

Efamol supplements have been used in a number of weight reduction trials involving obese individuals with successful results.

Amino acid supplements

Human growth hormone (HGH), produced by the pituitary gland in the brain, plays several vital roles in human metabolism, including the combustion of fat and its conversion into energy and muscle. This HGH is released by the body in response to exercise, fasting and sleep — peak secretion is reached about 90 minutes after we doze off.

After the age of 30, we tend to produce human growth hormone in smaller quantities. This partly accounts for many people's tendency to put on weight during middle age, despite eating no more than they did as teenagers.

Two amino acids, L-arginine and L-ornithine, stimulate the production and release of HGH and it has been suggested that these supplements can convert a normal 65-year-old's HGH levels into those resembling the levels in a young adult. A third amino acid, L-carnitine, (i.e. carnitine — see above) also plays a vital role in converting stored body fat into energy, by transferring fatty acids into the cells' mitochondria to be used as fuel. Dietary supplements of these amino acids have been shown to aid weight reduction by converting excessive body fat into lean muscular tissue.

Slim-Nite (Reevecrest Health Care Ltd), taken at bedtime on an empty stomach with juice or water or other non-protein drink, can help an overall weight reduction programme, provided it is based upon a sensible nutritious calorie-reduced dietary regimen. The recommended dose is three tablets before retiring to bed and the supplement is generally suitable for most would-be reducers, apart from those suffering from diabetes, herpes, or schizophrenia.

Do not take it if you are pregnant or below the age of 18.

CHAPTER 7

Easy exercise

Many people — especially those of us who could best make use of it — remain unconvinced of the value of regular physical exercise. The prospect of becoming more active can seem depressing and daunting, especially when we already feel overtired at the end of a busy day in the home or at work.

Driving in congested cities, travelling on public transport, shopping, housework, and looking after small children, often in addition to hours spent in an office, factory, or other place of employment, can make us too exhausted even to learn to relax! So it is little wonder that exercise is generally at the bottom of the list of health measures we are prepared to introduce into our daily lifestyle.

Nevertheless, exercise is proving a key factor in the treatment of both hypertension and cardiovascular disease. Monitored exercise is the key to the high success rate of the Cardiovascular Rehabilitation Centre at Houston, Texas. During its first seven years (1978–85), the Centre treated more than 1,000 patients, all of whom had been seriously ill, and about half of whom began treatment at risk of sudden death at any moment.

According to a report by David Loshat in GP (21st June 1985) 10 out of 12 patients who were waiting for heart transplant operations regained sufficiently good health to permit them to return to work and a normal life. The Centre's director and founder, Dr Lysle Peterson, former President of the International Cardiological Society, found that all the patients treated had improved their heart condition by 300 per cent regardless of their age. In addition, their use of diuretic, vasodilator, and beta blocker drugs had fallen by an overall 63 per cent.

All treatment is carried out at the Centre on a day-patient basis, and a rehabilitation course lasts for around 14 weeks, comprising two hours a day three times weekly. Not only is this form of treatment far more cost-effective, but it also achieves better effects than surgery and medication, although these still play a part in the management of a number of individuals.

The Centre uses a stationary exercise bicycle, since this provides a simple method of providing precisely the amount of exercise a patient needs, and for monitoring his or her heart beat and blood pressure. While jogging, squash, etc. can be dangerous for heart patients, stationary cycling at a predetermined therapeutic level has never resulted in the need to resuscitate a single patient, despite some of them being over 88 years old.

The effects of exercise

Healthy exercise training works on the overload principle. That is, you need to make only a little greater effort when performing it than that to which you are already accustomed. Two swimming-bath lengths of the crawl stroke may be sufficient for you in the early stages if you are unfit, whereas 40–50 lengths may be needed at a faster pace for a competitive swimmer. If you are not used to walking for many minutes at a time, 20–30 minutes spent walking briskly at around 3 mph will produce beneficial physiological and biochemical changes.

These include extra oxygen being extracted by the muscles of the body from the blood, and a reduced demand upon the heart muscle. Your resting heart rate becomes lower, and, when exercising, you will find your heart beating less rapidly than before, although it retains the full strength of its beat and output of blood. The muscles become more adept at extracting available oxygen, so less oxygenated, arterial blood is required to reach them. This means that when you really have to exert yourself unexpectedly, the effects upon your physiological processes and cardiovascular system will be far less drastic. In addition, once the heart starts to contract more effectively at each beat, and the rate at which it beats is reduced, the heart's muscle is spared much unnecessary work. These mechanisms help to explain the beneficial effects of exercise on the heart and blood vessels, and on other bodily systems.

Benefits of exercise

In an article which appeared in *The Practitioner* (December 1987, Vol. 231), entitled 'Reasons for Advising Exercise', the authors, Joan Bassey, Peter Fentem, and Nancy Turnbull of the Department of Physiology and Pharmacology, Queens Medical Centre, Nottingham, underline the advantages of regular exercise under several headings. Significantly, regular, increased physical activity seems to inhibit the rise in blood pressure, and reduce the frequency of arterial hypertension in previously healthy men and women as they grow older.

They say:

> In several intervention studies, adults with mild/moderate or labile systematic arterial hypertension . . . showed an average reduction of 13/10 millimetres Hg in arterial blood pressure with regular, moderate, endurance exercise. Hypertensive adolescents, and severely hypertensive women also showed reductions. This reduction in blood pressure may represent one mechanism by which physical activity contributes to the prevention of coronary heart disease and stroke.

Coronary heart disease

There is a proven direct relationship between regular, physical exercise and a healthy heart. Exercise that makes a demand upon the heart (aerobic exercise) increases its strength in the ways described above, and reduces the major known risk factors to coronary heart disease. Besides reducing blood pressure, it lowers the blood fat level, discourages clot formation (thrombosis), helps maintain a normal body weight, and releases emotional tension.

The importance of the last-mentioned factor is reflected in the 'Type A' personality profile which has been shown to be associated with a higher than normal risk of suffering a heart attack. Type A people tend to react badly to stress, become tense and frequently irritable, and characteristically worry about trivia; they also tend to be perfectionists, and 'high achievers'. Regular exercise is of particular benefit to people of this type, since it offers an opportunity for a release of their pent-up energy and tension.

While regular, monitored exercise cannot replace damaged

heart tissue with new, living cells following a coronary thrombosis, its overall benefits are felt by the rest of the healthy heart muscle. Recovery after a heart attack, when exercise is used as part of the treatment regimen, is normally more rapid and more successful, and the resultant feeling of getting back to 'normal' helps to relieve the melancholic forebodings from which many heart attack patients suffer.

Claudication

Doctors also recommend daily regular exercise for the treatment of arterial problems in other body areas. Diseased arteries in the legs cause cramping pain and a limp (claudication) when walking, because the leg muscles' extra demand for oxygen and nutrients is failing to be met by the diminished blood supply. While arterial surgery can 'declog' and sometimes replace sections of diseased peripheral arteries, many physicians and vascular surgeons now prefer the more conservative approach of a carefully controlled, gradually-increasing walking regimen. Regular leg exercise of this type, carried out by many scores of patients, has proved highly beneficial, since it has been found to result in the growth of new blood vessels in the affected leg muscles. This results in patients being able to walk further and further, without claudication symptoms, over a period of weeks or months.

Osteoporosis

Exercise also helps to combat the bone-thinning disease, osteoporosis. All adults lose calcium from their bones from around the age of 35 onwards, but the condition is particularly serious in women, who lose considerably more than men in their late 40s and early 50s when the menopause takes place and their blood oestrogen levels fall. Osteoporotic bones become brittle and fracture easily. The most serious fracture affecting elderly women is that of the neck of the femur (the upper end of the long thigh bone as it enters the hip joint): 15 per cent of patients with this injury die within three months, and the condition costs the National Health Service in excess of £100 million annually.

Diabetes

Diabetics run an increased risk of developing diseased, fat-clogged arteries and other vascular problems. Exercise proves useful in this capacity since it improves a tolerance of carbohydrates and increases the body cells' sensitivity to whatever insulin the pancreas is able to produce.

Insomnia

A further bonus is the promotion of sound, healthy sleep. The demands of a busy, stressful lifestyle make adequate rest imperative, yet many exhausted individuals lie awake night after night, tossing, turning and fretting about daily worries which inevitably become magnified out of all proportion in the dark, small hours. Chronic insomnia can have an adverse effect on many aspects of health, and can put the thought of daily physical exertion out of the question.

Paradoxically, aerobic or 'demand' exercise tires you healthily;

Table 2: The effect of exercise on heart disease high risk factors

Blood pressure	
Systolic	↓ 13 mm HG
Diastolic	↓ 10 mm HG
Blood fat levels (lipoproteins)	
Healthy lipoproteins	↑
Harmful lipoproteins	↓
Total cholesterol	↓
Triglycerides	↓
Clotting factors	
Anticlotting function	↑
Proclotting function	↓ (After vigorous exercise)
Metabolism	
Energy balance regulation	↑
Heart	
Heart muscle work	↓
Risk of irregular rhythms	↓
Heart rate	↓

following it, tense, taut muscles relax, and a regular sleep pattern can often be re-established without the use of drugs.

How to start

The best approach is to aim at taking regular exercise; for example, three 20–30 minute exercise sessions every week. The worst approach is to take up a very demanding sport such as squash, spend out on new clothes and equipment, and rush at your new project with unbridled enthusiasm when you haven't exercised for years. At best, you are likely to become rapidly exhausted and disillusioned, and give up exercising as quickly as you started, perhaps suffering a tendon, joint, or soft tissue injury into the bargain. You may do yourself serious harm, and at worst, if you're very unfit and suffering from high blood pressure, may even bring on the heart attack you are seeking to avert.

Your choice of exercise should be based on two considerations. Most importantly, it should be a form of activity which you are likely to enjoy. Secondly, it should involve rhythmic action which makes use of the body's large muscle groups. Brisk walking and swimming are ideal. If you cannot swim, now is the time to learn. You may claim to dislike walking, and it is often an unpleasant experience when confined to hard pavements, and busy, polluted streets. However, most urban areas are close to a park, common or open space, so buy some comfortable, good quality trainers, don a tracksuit or other loose comfortable clothing, and set out to become regularly acquainted with your local sample of the countryside.

The secret is to start modestly, and a further helpful hint is to avoid telling all and sundry of your new exercise scheme. Even well-meaning people frequently ridicule the health measures which they are not prepared to follow themselves, and sensing safety in numbers, they feel ill at ease until you relinquish your aims and rejoin their ranks.

Ask your doctor to check your heart and blood pressure first, before taking up exercise, if these have ever presented problems. Set yourself small goals initially, starting with 5–10 minutes of gentle exercise, and building up in gradual stages until you are well able to tolerate a full half hour of aerobic activity.

Do not confine exercise to your thrice-weekly training sessions. Start living more actively right away by climbing stairs instead of taking the lift, gradually increasing the storeys you walk up in a tall building. Take additional short walks wherever possible — if you normally get the car out to take a short trip to the newsagents or local shops, try leaving it behind! Join in with your children's or grandchildren's sports and games. Hopefully they'll be delighted at your participation, and you, and they, may learn a lot!

Always limber up for five minutes before and after an exercise session. Rotate your shoulder joints, gently flex your arm, wrist, hip, knee, and ankle joints, and shake your arms about, loosening up your fingers. Try to touch your toes — and don't be dismayed if this is impossible. One of the benefits of your exercise regimen will soon show itself to be improved joint and muscle flexibility.

Table 3: Exercising pulse rates by age and fitness

Age	Max heart rate	Exercise pulse rate (unfit)	Exercise pulse rate (fit)
16	204	123	164
18	202	122	162
20	200	120	160
22	198	119	158
24	196	118	157
26	194	116	155
28	192	115	154
30	190	114	152
32	188	113	150
34	186	112	149
36	184	110	147
38	182	109	146
40	180	108	144
45	175	105	140
50	170	102	136
55	165	99	132
60	160	96	128
65	155	93	124
70	150	90	120
75	145	87	116
80	140	84	112

Finally, run slowly and gently on the spot. The following table shows the pulse rates at which to aim when exercising, according to your age and fitness. Refer to the higher of two ages, if you are between them. *Do not aim* to reach your maximum heart rate (second column). This figure is used to calculate the level to which your pulse should rise for you to benefit, and is calculated by subtracting your age in years from 220. Your pulse rate should reach 60 per cent of the maximum heart rate if you are unfit, and 80 per cent if you are fit.

As you will see, the age column extends from 16 to 80 years. According to a report in *Geriatric Medicine* (May 1986), only a proportion of decline in elderly people results from the disease process; much of it is caused by underuse. For a variety of reasons, including stiffness, pain and weakness, elderly people make less use of a particular part of their body and become less active, in this way widening the gap between possible and actual fitness. Oxford Community Physician, J.A. Muir Gray, pointed out in the report that many veterans' sporting records demonstrate that the loss of fitness due to age alone is a great deal less than most people, including many doctors, would imagine.

'There is every reason to encourage people to try to keep fit as they grow older as a way of preventing some of the problems typical of old age', said Dr Muir Gray. He referred to encouraging evidence which suggests that fitness can be regained in old age: in one study, seven weeks' conditioning improved oxygen-demanding power activity by 30 per cent, and 'maximum oxygen intake was brought quite quickly to the level anticipated in a sedentary person ten to twenty years younger than the test subject'. Other research studies suggest that suppleness, strength, and skill, in addition to stamina, can be significantly improved in elderly people.

The following table appeared in *Geriatric Medicine* (May 1986):

Table 4: Fit veterans' peak performance is surprisingly close to that of their younger counterparts (British Veterans' cycling records, 1983)

25 miles		50 miles		100 miles	
Age	Time	Age	Time	Age	Time
43	52.45	43	1.47.38	43	3.51.25
66	57.05	66	2.52.41	66	4.16.37
77	1.08.00	77	2.19.57	76	5.16.53
82	1.37.00	78	2.52.38		

CHAPTER 8

Relaxation techniques

As we saw during the earlier discussion upon the effects of stress, prolonged tension and worry, combined with adverse factors in our social and/or domestic environment, increase the release of the stress hormones adrenaline and noradrenaline into the bloodstream. This process is in fact just one highly important aspect of a wide spectrum of neurophysiological processes triggered by stress, and resulting from stimulation of the autonomic nervous system.

As its name applies, the autonomic nervous system functions outside our conscious control. It regulates bodily functions such as our heartbeat, respiration, hormone release and the multitude of physiological and biochemical processes which continue to function independently of any effort that we can make, day and night, throughout our entire lives.

This part of our nervous system functions by reflex action. The majority of bodily functions are controlled in this way, including the dilation and constriction of blood vessels in the skin in response to external temperature change, the constriction of the pupils of the eye to bright light, and the production of saliva immediately before, and during, eating.

The autonomic nervous system comprises two discrete sets of nerves. Many organs, blood vessels and glands receive nerve fibres from both, their function being regulated by the balance of their opposed activity. Sympathetic nerves arise from small collections of nerve cells called ganglia, found in pairs throughout the greater part of the spinal cord. Messages from the brain to the sympathetic ganglia generate impulses in sympathetic nerve fibres, generally resulting in the release of adrenaline and nor-adrenaline in the parts of the body and tissues that they supply.

and tissues that they supply.

While the function of the sympathetic nervous system is closely related to blood pressure increase, its counterpart, the parasympathetic nervous system, has the reverse effect. Parasympathetic nerves arise in the body in two main groups. The most important of these, the vagus nerve, arises from the base of the brain, travels down among the structures of the neck to the thorax (chest) where it sends off branches to the heart, and travels downwards through the diaphragm into the abdomen where it sends vital branches to the stomach, increasing, among other factors, the secretion of hydrochloric acid during the process of digestion.

The second portion of the parasympathetic nervous system arises from the lower end of the spinal cord, and is intimately connected with the function of the bladder and other pelvic organs. In contrast to the sympathetic nervous system, the parasympathetic functions by releasing the neurotransmitter chemical messenger, acetylcholine, from its terminal nerve endings.

Besides transferring messages from the brain and central nervous system, the autonomic nerves also relay sensation from the bodily organs to the brain. In some instances, these result in reflex effects in appropriate bodily areas, and do not reach our conscious awareness. A rise in blood pressure, for instance, reaches the brain and results in nerve stimuli travelling by the vagus parasympathetic nerves to the heart muscle, to decrease its activity. The fact that many high blood pressure sufferers have a fast pulse rate in addition to hypertension reflects the fact that their sympathetic nerves are currently in 'overdrive', i.e. they are overriding the beneficial effects of the parasympathetic nerves. Certain autonomic nervous system messages *do* reach conscious awareness. A sudden shock, accident, or unpleasant sight can send alarm messages racing through our autonomic nervous system, which result in immediate nausea and vomiting. In this case, awareness of sympathetic/parasympathetic activity is both strong and unpleasant.

Harnessing parasympathetic power

Many modern psychologically orientated therapies, especially those stemming from the United States, have over the past 15 years urged us to get into contact with our 'inner selves' by a variety of means. While increased insight into our mental make-up and the way our bodies function is largely to be applauded, some proponents of 'getting in touch' techniques go overboard in their enthusiasm. The suggestions made in this book for getting in touch with your parasympathetic nervous system are urbane and, above all, practicable.

Parasympathetic activity counteracts the sympathetic nervous system processes that are largely responsible for generating high blood pressure. While sympathetic activity can best be visualized by imagining yourself in a 'flight or fight' situation, with tense muscles, dilated pupils, a rapid heart beat, quick shallow breathing and some of your hairs literally standing on end, parasympathetic activity can best be understood by imagining yourself asleep in an armchair after a large lunch.

In this instance, your body's main need is to divert extra blood to your stomach and bowel, to aid the process of digestion. The muscles of your arms, legs, and trunk are loose and relaxed; your eyelids are closed, your pupils constricted, your heartbeat normal to slow, and your breathing even, deep and regular. Moreover, instead of large quantities of adrenaline and noradrenaline pouring into your blood stream from your adrenal glands, your body's main hormonal concern is directed towards the release of digestive enzymes in response to your meal. Most important, in the present context, your blood pressure is normal or as low as it is likely to get if you already suffer from hypertension.

Doctors and other health experts have coined the term trophotropic to describe the response of the parasympathetic nervous system. Its activities are those of slowing, tranquillizing, and inhibiting sympathetic activity, and restoring both mind and body to a state of balance and harmony. Relaxation techniques produce this condition, and are increasingly used by both doctors and alternative practitioners since deep relaxation has been found highly conducive to positive health. Conditions known to benefit include tachycardia (a fast heart beat), palpitations, and high blood pressure, together with a wide spectrum of anxiety symptoms, so often found in association with hypertension. These include sleep problems, irritability and tension, fatigue, exhaustion and reactive depression. Other related symptoms comprise hyperventilation (rapid breathing), nausea, shakiness, panic attacks, phobias, dizziness, migraine, asthma, and premenstrual syndrome (PMS).

In her feature 'The Use of Relaxation Techniques in General Practice', Julienne McLean M.Sc., Medical Psychologist at the Department of General Practice, St Mary's Hospital Medical School, London, discusses neuromuscular relaxation and meditation in the treatment of high blood pressure and other conditions, as described below.

Neuromuscular relaxation

This relaxation method reduces tension and nerve activity in the muscles of the body under our conscious control. Progressive muscular relaxation, developed by Edmund Jacobson, is a popular form. Jacobson emphasizes the value of the individual learning the difference between tension and relaxation, and his method consists of the contraction, followed by the relaxation, of selected muscles and muscle groups throughout the body. A state of deep relaxation follows the treatment of all the main body muscles in this manner. Some therapists advocate contracting and relaxing several muscle groups at a time, e.g. the left leg, arm and side of the abdomen, while others favour working up the body from feet to skull contracting smaller muscle groups in a more systematic way. Thus, the subject may be instructed first to contract and relax the muscles of the left foot, noting the sensations, and to follow this by repeating the exercise with the right foot.

Some practitioners prefer to use a passive rather than a physically active form of relaxation. The basis of this variation is getting the patient to focus his or her attention on a series of individual muscle groups, and then relaxing them through a process of direct concentration. Here, the use of mental imagery is important, the patient being asked to visualize, for example, and then feel — i.e. be aware of — the muscles of the left calf, thigh, abdomen etc.

It has been suggested that anxiety can be split into thought-orientated and body-orientated forms, localized in the two hemispheres of the brain, and that different forms of relaxation are appropriate for different types of anxiety. Two researchers, Davidson and Schwartz (1976), who have delved deeply into the subject, have suggested that progressive muscular relaxation is the most effective form of treatment for body-orientated anxiety.

It has been found highly effective in the treatment of essential hypertension, sleep problems, migraine, tension headaches, and other aspects of anxiety, including psychosomatic pain. Sometimes, other forms of treatment for a patient's stress need to include behaviour therapy or other forms of psychotherapy as adjuncts to relaxation.

Meditation

In her discussion of this subject, Julienne McLean points out that although it has been used for thousands of years 'within the religious and philosophical traditions of the east', only for the past 30 years has it been used as a form of medical and psychotherapeutic treatment without religious connotations. All meditation techniques make use of a focal device, upon which the individual concentrates his or her attention. This may be a visual image, such as a mandala, or a flower; physical activity such as dancing, breathing or jogging; or mental repetition, such as a mantra, prayer or chant. Euphonious, flowing words should be chosen with care for their suitability to the individual patient, and phrases involving several words should have a positive, confidence-boosting meaning.

Meditation brings about the trophotropic state, by encouraging the intuitive type of thought pattern characteristic of the brain's right hemisphere to predominate in the individual's consciousness rather than of the usually dominant, analytical thought mode, progressing from the left hemisphere. Physiological changes reported to take place during meditation include slowing of the heart rate, a reduced oxygen consumption, decreased respiration rate, an increased regularity of alpha brain wave activity, and a reduction in blood pressure. These responses are not unique to meditation, it is now believed, but common to all passive relaxation techniques. Research studies into the use of meditation in reducing high blood pressure have consistently shown a reduction in blood pressure in the treatment group, a reduction in the use of antihypertensive drugs, and a reduction in bodily symptoms. Follow-up data have shown that treatment gains were maintained over a twelve-month period and also after four years.

Biofeedback training

Biofeedback training is a method of monitoring bodily functions, and using information gained about them to bring about necessary and desirable changes. Our bodies utilize the principle of feedback in order to operate as an integral whole. The sympathetic nervous system uses it, when we are subjected to stress. Emotions such as fear or excitement, arising in the cortex of the brain, send stimuli to the hypothalamus in the mid-brain, which in turn helps to generate impulses in the sympathetic nervous system. In this example of biofeedback, data from the brain's emotional centres is 'fed' to the hypothalamus, which utilizes it to set in motion the necessary sympathetic response.

Biofeedback calls into action a function of the human mind that has been explored most fully in the past by the use of hypnotism. Hypnosis has been used experimentally to cause a number of bodily changes such as an increase in skin temperature, and the disappearance of rashes, warts etc. It works by harnessing the power of the subconscious mind while the individual is in a hypnotic trance. Biofeedback is now used to give people a high degree of control over physiological events that were once throught to be outside conscious control. Biofeedback training seems to make nonsense of the statement made earlier in this chapter that the autonomic nervous system governs those bodily functions outside the control of the conscious mind. The contradiction is only a partial one, however.

Biofeedback training has been used in Western medicine for around 30 years, and hundreds of papers have been written about its use. In practical terms, it is carried out by the doctor or therapist attaching the patient to some kind of electronic or electrical apparatus, which monitors a particular output from a bodily system, and displays the results in such a way, visibly or audibly, that the person can keep a constant tab on the success of his efforts. If, for example, he is asked to 'try to relax', successful achievement of this task may be reflected by a loud hum, or a row of coloured lights. It is difficult to tell a person how to relax, so biofeedback training marshals a person's innate awareness of how this is done. It is very difficult indeed to try to explain, for example, how to ride a bicycle. This can only be learned by the method of trial and error, and involves practising to the point at which you 'get the feel' of the degree of balance and muscular co-ordination required. One method uses a galvanic skin response (GSR) device which picks up tiny quantities of perspiration on the skin of the subject's fingertips. The greater the state of tension, the greater the perspiration output. As the tension is replaced by a more relaxed state, less perspiration is produced, thereby acquainting the person with what has to be done in order to achieve tranquility of mind and body.

In an instance such as this, no complicated instructions are given. Subjects undergoing the training usually starts by relaxing their bodily muscles, only to discover that success is partial, i.e. the machine is producing a hum at half its normal pitch, or only some of the coloured lights on the machine have lit up. They then generally try out the effects of different frames of mind. This could include visualizing a restful scene such as a beach or a woodland glade, or imagining oneself surrounded by a bubble of clear blue light. What works for one individual is usually peculiar to him or her, and may not be effective for another subject.

Excellent results have been obtained using biofeedback training in combination with yoga, meditation, and other specific relaxation techniques. Doctors Chandra Patel and W.R.S. North reported the results of a study in *The Lancet* (19 July 1975). Working with 34 patients suffering from high blood pressure, they organized two forms of treatment to which the patients were randomly assigned — one was a 'placebo' therapy consisting of general relaxation, and the other was a combination of yoga relaxation methods and biofeedback training.

Both groups showed a reduction in blood pressure, after the six-week period. The average reading of the general relaxation group was reduced from 169/101 to 160/96 mm Hg, while the biofeedback/yoga group showed an average reduction from 168/100 to 141/84 mm Hg. Statistically, a fall of 16 mm Hg in diastolic blood pressure is extremely significant.

Doctors North and Patel used Jacobson's progressive relaxation techniques, discussed above, in the first instance, and then taught the relevant patients transcendental meditation. To increase the success of both methods, each patient involved was connected to two biofeedback machines giving a continuous audio signal whose pitch fell as relaxation was achieved. The first machine was a GSR device, and the second was a machine which measured electrical activity in muscles.

The doctors said in their report:

Patients were also encouraged verbally and were shown their blood pressure records; they were also instructed to practise relaxation and meditation twice a day, and gradually to try to incorporate these habits into routine activities, the methods depending upon individual circumstances. For example, each patient had a red disc attached to his watch to remind him to relax whenever he looked at the time, and some were told to relax before answering the telephone.

Many doctors feel that biofeedback equipment should be used only under professional supervision. Training devices are offered for sale to the public, and most intelligent people can use such a machine successfully in order to teach themselves how to relax. However, it is most important to get medical advice before undertaking biofeedback training as a form of treatment.

CHAPTER 9

Cigarettes, alcohol and hypertension

Many would-be non-smokers believe that there is a secret which, if they learned, would enable them to quit their habit successfully. This is true, and the secret is so simple that most people overlook it. It is no more, and no less, than actually *wanting* to quit the habit badly enough to make the effort.

The majority of smokers give up at some point in their lives — and some do so many times over. But frequently, the withdrawal symptoms from nicotine, and the loss of a long-established and familiar habit, cause them to restart. Smokers who do give up permanently achieve their goal just because they are determined to do so at all costs. If you have tried and failed, facing the facts about cigarettes, high blood pressure, and premature death should help to give you the necessary willpower.

Cigarettes and your body

All cigarette packets bear a warning along the lines that their contents can cause lung cancer, bronchitis and other chest diseases. If packets of biscuits or sweets bearing a similar message, were introduced into the shops, there would be a public outcry. As it is, sales of cigarettes, tobacco and cigars continue, despite a fall over the past five years.

Everyone knows that cigarettes can cause lung cancer, but few are aware of their close link with heart disease, heart attacks, and hypertension. A list of high risk factors predisposing people to cardiovascular disease, based on data drawn from research studies, confirms that cigarette smoking is among the most important of them. Hundreds of clinical trials and aetiological studies have confirmed that there is little doubt about the predictive power of these factors. Estimates based on the Framingham Heart Study and national statistics show us that two out of every three deaths from heart attacks and diseased coronary arteries happen to people exposed to them.

As specialist Robert I. Levy says in 'Prevalence and Epidemiology of Cardiovascular Disease' in Cecil's *Textbook Of Medicine*, edited by James B. Wyngaarden MD and Lloyd H. Smith (Jnr) MD,

> Cigarette smoking has clearly been shown to be an independent, potent risk factor for coronary, cerebral and peripheral vascular disease. Sudden cardiac death, heart attack, angina, claudication, and stroke incidence and prevalence can be related to the number of cigarettes one smokes. The heavier the cigarette smoking history, the higher the risk.

As explained in Chapter 3, peripheral vascular disease has a close association with the development of high blood pressure.

Dr Levy continues:

> Both nicotine and carbon monoxide inhaled with cigarette smoking have been incriminated as causative factors, but definite understanding of cause and effect still eludes us . . . Furthermore, in contrast to the apparently accumulative relationship of cigarette smoking to lung cancer, a series of prospective and retrospective studies now indicates that if one stops smoking cigarettes, *over 90 per cent of the increased cardiovascular risk disappears within eighteen months* [my italics].

This very encouraging fact should make the effort of quitting smoking worthwhile.

One of the means by which cigarette smoking increases blood pressure is by accelerating the development of atherosclerotic arterial disease. The increased risk of this is plainly shown in the increased incidence of heart attacks, strokes and intermittent claudication seen in smokers — with peripheral vascular disease being the main risk to women. By the age of 45, male smokers run a 70 per cent increased risk of serious disease and death.

Up to the time of the menopause, women receive a certain

amount of protection against heart disease and coronary thrombosis from their sex hormones. As their oestrogen levels start to decline (this begins well before menopausal symptoms start) they lose this protection, and over the past 15 years heart attacks have increased by 10 per cent in women as opposed to 3 per cent in men.

Significantly, although fewer women now smoke, the rate of smokers among teenage girls has increased and women smokers smoke more heavily than was once the case. As well as favouring blocked, fatty arteries and hypertension, smoking brings on the menopause at an earlier age, thereby hastening the removal of protective oestrogen.

A further effect is an increase in free radical activity in the bodily tissues. Free radicals are electrically charged fragments of molecules produced during normal cellular biochemical processes but capable, when produced in excess, of causing severe tissue damage. Stress (see Chapter 8), atmospheric pollution, and other toxic substances also increase free radical manufacture. Among their adverse effects, these molecular fragments increase the risk of degenerative disease such as arthritis and cancer, speed up the ageing process, and impair the strength of the immune defence system.

Ironically, vitamin C is a potent fighter of free radical activity, and it is this very vitamin that smoking destroys. In fact, you lose about 25 mg vitamin C for every cigarette you consume.

In addition to tar, cigarette smoke contains over two thousand chemicals, many of which enter the bloodstream through the respiratory surface of the lungs and have a direct effect on vital body organs, including the brain, heart and blood vessels.

Nicotine

Smokers claim that cigarettes 'calm their nerves'. Some studies show that nicotine has a relaxing effect upon body and limb muscles, but its effects upon the central nervous system is excitatory. It enhances the activity of certain enzymes in the liver, where it is largely metabolized, in this way increasing its own rate of breakdown. This accounts, in part, for the development of tolerance to its effects, resulting in the need for an increased number of cigarettes daily.

Nicotine also stimulates the adrenal glands, enhancing their output of the stress hormone adrenaline. This increases sympathetic nervous activity, including the constriction of peripheral blood vessels leading decreased body temperature and increased blood pressure.

Carbon monoxide

Present in some commercial gases and produced by the combustion of petrol, this substance is potentially lethal. Suicide resulting from breathing car exhaust fumes results from carbon monoxide poisoning. It affects the haemoglobin (coloured pigment) present in red blood cells, which is responsible for transporting oxygen around the body from the lungs to the tissues and organs.

Under normal conditions, the oxygen we breathe in attaches itself to red cell haemoglobin, forming a compound called oxyhaemoglobin. The bonds between the oxygen and the pigment are loose, and oxygen is readily released in the tissues when necessary.

Carbon monoxide interferes with this process by attaching itself to haemoglobin in place of the oxygen, forming a tightly bonded compound called methoxyhaemoglobin. Death results largely from oxygen starvation.

Cigarettes and your brain

While no specific link has yet been proven between cigarette smoking and brain damage similar to that involving alcohol, there is no doubt that the general effects of inhaled cigarette smoke on brain cells are adverse. The brain's oxygen requirement is both high and constant, and clogged cerebral (brain) arteries eventually carry a lower supply of oxygenated blood to the various areas of the brain as atherosclerotic disease progresses. They also become especially prone to damage and clot formation, leading to cerebral haemorrhage and stroke.

Psychologically, many smokers find difficulty in abandoning their habit because cigarettes 'give them something to do with their hands'. Unlikely as this may seem to non-smokers, who unconsciously rely on other body language strategies to give themselves confidence, this can present a major problem to many. Relaxation methods (see Chapter 8) are the best solution.

Cigarette smoking — how to stop

Chewing gum containing nicotine has been available for some years in the UK, Europe and the United States. It can help you give up the habit of smoking, while dampening the withdrawal symptoms from addictive nicotine. Some reports of this therapy show promising results, and the side-effects, which include hiccups, mouth and tongue irritation, and heartburn, are generally mild.

A variety of aversion techniques exists. These are based on behaviour modification ideas, stemming from behavioural psychology, and link the act of smoking with an unpleasant experience. Electric aversion therapy, which many practitioners claim to have a high success rate, applies non-dangerous, although unpleasant, electric shocks to the patient during treatment sessions while he smokes. The idea is that the patient soon links smoking with an unacceptable physical experience, and rapidly grows to dislike it. The technique is easy to carry out, generally inexpensive — at least so far as equipment is concerned — and readily controlled by the therapist.

Rapid smoking therapy involves the patient smoking his or her favourite brand of cigarettes very quickly, at around one puff every six seconds, until he or she can no longer continue. The treatment room is usually decorated with cigarette advertisements, and contains several ashtrays overflowing with offensively smelling cigarette ash and butts. Sometimes electric shocks are administered as well, although many therapists feel that this is unnecessary.

Many studies have shown rapid smoking therapy to have a high success rate, but it can be dangerous to health. It leads to a high blood level of both nicotine and carboxyhaemoglobin (see Carbon monoxide, p.107), which many experts feel make it unsuitable for smokers other than the young and healthy. It is particularly risky for people with clogged coronary arteries and anyone over 35, who may have an existing but undiagnosed heart condition.

Hypnotherapy is also useful. Some hypnotherapists use an aversion technique while the patient is in a state of trance, suggesting to the subconscious mind that cigarettes will henceforth taste of something particularly unpleasant. Others rely more upon ego boosting, i.e. confidence building, getting the message through to the patient's subconscious mind that he or she will from then on feel relaxed rather than tense in stressful situations, when socializing etc, and that the need to smoke will rapidly diminish. Some therapists succeed with a single consultation and hypnotherapy session only.

Others use the 'Q-day' technique. This consists of four hypnotherapy/counselling sessions, usually at seven-day intervals, during which cigarette consumption is reduced by an amount mutually agreed between therapist and patient until Q-day, that is quitting day, is reached, by the final session.

You may need some kind of therapeutic aid to quit smoking. On the other hand, you may decide to 'go it alone'. Rather than trying to reinforce your willpower which can lead to increased tension, an increased need for cigarettes, and failure, master a relaxation technique before you stop, and damp down sympathetic nervous activity under stressful conditions, particularly when withdrawal symptoms are getting to you, by putting the technique into practice. It is also helpful to set aside the money you normally waste on cigarettes every week, and use it to offset outstanding bills which anyway increase your tension or, if possible, save it up for a special treat for you, your partner or family.

Alcohol and high blood pressure

A number of studies have indicated that heavy drinking is a significant risk factor in the development of high blood pressure. INTERSALT, an international study involving more than 10,000 men and women from 52 centres, examined the association between alcohol intake and blood pressure in addition to body mass index and various biochemical parameters. It turned out that, on average, people drinking more than three to four units daily had a systolic blood pressure of 3.5 mm Hg higher than that of non-drinkers. As Professor Michael Marmot told delegates at a meeting of the British Hypertensive Society in Edinburgh in Autumn 1988, a 5 mm Hg reduction in blood pressure throughout the population as a whole would be associated with a 10–12 per cent decrease in the death rate from heart and blood vessel disease.

Alcohol and your body

Besides generating high blood pressure, alcohol abuse leads to other cardiovascular problems. These include heart palpitations, abnormal heart rhythms and sudden death, and chronic damage to the muscle of the heart leading to an increasing degree of heart failure.

Alcohol abuse also affects other bodily systems. It causes fatty infiltration of the liver, hepatitis, cirrhosis and eventual liver failure, and the formation of liver tumours (hepatoma). It affects the stomach and intestinal system by causing irritation to the stomach lining (gastritis), diarrhoea, disease of the pancreas, poor food absorption, and overweight; and it increases the risk of cancer of the food pipe (oesophagus). Heavy drinkers also run an increased risk of lung disease, especially chemical pneumonia, due to inhalation of vomit when in an alcoholic stupor. Alcohol abuse in women leads to sexual problems, irregular periods, and shrinkage of breasts and the external genitals; in men, it can cause loss of sex drive, reduced potency, a reduced or absent sperm count and infertility, and shrinkage of the penis and testes.

Alcohol and your brain

Alcohol abuse can inflict persistent brain damage. Various parts of the brain can degenerate, leading to dementia, and it increases the risk of brain blood vessel disease, including bleeding episodes (subarachnoid haemorrhage), strokes — especially in young people — and the formation of blood clots in the brain following head injury.

Other effects on the nervous system include weakness, paralysis, and tingling/pins and needles in the hands and feet. Withdrawal symptoms include fits, hallucinations, and trembling of the hands.

Psychiatric illness is common in alcohol abusers. Anxiety neurosis, and severe depression are common, as are loss of memory (amnesia), and sleeping problems. Depression, suicidal tendencies, anxiety, and insomnia bring in their wake problems at work and home. Rows, physical and verbal violence, absenteeism, inefficiency, loss of interest in everyday affairs and relationships, and divorce also commonly result.

What constitutes abuse?

A unit of alcohol is defined in standard units, where one unit is equivalent to half a pint of beer, a four-ounce glass of table wine, a glass of sherry, or a single whisky, gin or other form of spirits. Social drinkers are usually defined as people who drink no more than two to three units of alcohol daily, don't become intoxicated, and aren't likely to harm themselves or their family. Moderate drinkers regularly consume more than five units of alcohol a day, although apparently without immediate harm. The amount of alcohol we, as individuals, can take differs widely, with respect to its effects upon us and our lives, and problem drinkers are defined as people who experience physical, psychological, social, family, occupational, financial, or legal problems directly attributable to drinking, regardless of the amount.

Dependent drinkers consume roughly the same quantity of alcohol each day. Drinking is the most important factor in their lives, and many quit the habit only to resume it after a period of abstinence. They tend to have an increased tolerance to alcohol in the early stages of dependence, and reduced tolerance later on. They experience withdrawal symptoms when deprived of alcohol, which they relieve by drinking more.

Signs of dependence to watch out for include a growing preoccupation with alcohol, combined with defensiveness about consumption, early morning drinking, and the feeling of absolute necessity to get a drink. Character changes include increasing aggressiveness, denial and anger if tackled on the subject, and increasing absenteeism from work.

Young people, too, run a particularly high risk nowadays. In a recent survey reported in the *Guardian* (14 Dec. 1988), television commercials appear to reinforce under-age drinking, and more than 60 per cent of children/adolescents aged 10 to 17 were able to identify a minimum of four out of nine alcoholic drinks when they were shown still pictures from TV commercials. The advertising research unit from Strathclyde University found that up to 70 per cent recognized individual brands. The majority enjoyed drink commercials; only 31 per cent thought them boring, and 58 per cent opposed banning them.

Elderly people are not immune from the problem of alcohol. A recent UK survey showed that up to 30 per cent of the over-60s drink heavily enough to risk liver damage.

Who is at risk?

All but teetotallers run some risk of becoming alcohol abusers, and the safest advice to follow is to avoid alcohol when you are depressed, anxious, stressed, or tired. However much tension and fatigue may increase your desire to 'tipple', your body and brain can become used to the soothing effects of a glass of sherry, wine or beer far sooner than you may realize.

As a nation the British are drinking more than they were a decade ago, and over that period women in particular have increased their alcohol consumption.

How to stop excessive drinking

An alcohol abuser in the family is a sick person and requires urgent help, but the problems he or she can cause to other family members would be hard to exaggerate. The organization, Alateen, helps young people whose parents or close relations are alcohol dependent, while Al-Anon helps the families of alcoholics. For help and information about local branches, contact either of these at Family Groups UK and Eire, 61 Great Dover Street, Southwark, London SE1 4YF; tel. (01) 403 0888.

Some hospitals have special units and a number of private clinics offer medical treatment and counselling. Your GP should be able to give you the information you require about local facilities. The national drink watchers network, with branches throughout the country, offer advice and help on monitoring individual drinking patterns. The best-known organization, Alcoholics Anonymous, can be contacted at General Service Office, P.O. Box 1, Stonebow House, Stonebow, York YO1 2NJ. Tel. (0904) 644026/7/8/9. Alcohol Concern, based at 305 Gray's Inn Road, London WC1X 8QF, tel. (01) 833 3471, provides information about help with drinking problems available nationally and locally. In the USA, Alcoholics Anonymous are based at 468 Park Avenue South, New York, NY 10016; tel. (212) 686 1100. Elsewhere, check the Yellow Pages.

CHAPTER 10

Alternative therapies

Alternative (complementary) therapies are used increasingly in this country for a wide range of illnesses. The more commonly practised ones — acupuncture, homoeopathy, osteopathy, chiropractic — have been used in the UK and Europe for many years. But the 1970s and 1980s have seen a particularly notable growth in their acceptance and availability, and the orthodox medical profession are now referring patients to alternative practitioners and, in many cases, learning to practise some of the disciplines themselves.

Medical herbalism needs special mention. Not only has it been the main source of medical treatment for many millions of people both in Europe and other parts of the world since time immemorial; it has also provided the foundation upon which modern pharmaceutical knowledge has developed into a vital and highly sophisticated science.

However, much still remains to be understood about complementary therapies and their underlying philosophy. Many people remain sceptical about the value of piercing the skin of the ear lobe with an acupuncture needle, for example, in order to relieve food cravings and withdrawal symptoms from cigarette smoking. Homoeopathy is still ridiculed by those who, while not denying that like may well cure like, doubt that the potency of homoeopathic remedies is inversely proportional to the amount of active substance they contain. And reflexology — pressure applied to the soles of the feet at certain predetermined points — strikes many newcomers to alternative medicine as an odd way to relieve backache, peptic ulcer pain, or eczema.

The main thing to remember about alternative therapies is that they are based on an alternative view of how the body functions.

Conventional medicine sees disease in terms of direct cause and effect, and treats cystitis, for example, with antibiotics to kill bacteria, and a head cold with aspirin to relieve the fever and inflammation. Alternative practitioners, by contrast, take a broader, i.e. holistic, view and attribute illness to a disturbance in the overall harmony that exists in a healthy person, between body, mind, and spirit.

Alternative therapies aim to discover the reason for the causative imbalance and to redress it wherever possible. They recognize the existence of the life force, which they equate with the principle differentiating living from non-living matter, and state that its potency depends upon the harmony and the smooth co-operation of all those parts, physical and ethereal, of which we are composed. Although conventional medicine can offer specific treatments — in particular, drugs — for the vast majority of ailments, the alternatives, based upon a broader philosophy, use a relatively small number of corrective techniques.

The concept of the life force, and the rationale of manoeuvres to restore its strength, have been the focus of most of the controversy separating orthodox and complementary medicine. Yet with the advent of increasing evidence in support of the reality of the life force, and the success achieved by complementary therapists in cases where conventional medicine has failed, the dichotomy is being steadily bridged. Doctors who add acupuncture to the treatments they offer their patients may not think of this discipline in terms of freeing clogged channels (meridians) along which the life force flows, but the medical profession as a whole is paying increasing attention to objective scientific evidence supporting the interdependence of mind and body, and the possible adverse effects of one upon the other.

Alternative practitioners attribute great importance to the effects of the emotions on the human organism, and counselling plays a major role in many of their therapies. Traditionally, medical doctors set less store on talking and listening than upon prescribing medicines and tablets. Recent research has shown, however, that the immune defence system, our main means of protection against invading bacteria and viruses, malignant cell change, and premature ageing, is weakened by stress, anxiety and depression — and that we become more susceptible to both infectious illness and cancer when persistently tense and unhappy.

Circumstantial proof of this kind has already gone a long way towards emphasizing the vital interplay between body, mind and spirit. As research reveals further evidence of this nature, orthodox doctors will inevitably grow closer to an understanding and an acceptance of the alternative view. And, as in all balanced systems, there are advantages to both sides. Many complementary practitioners are coming to feel the need to base the therapies they practise upon a more scientific and disciplined basis. This does not mean that reflexology, for instance, lacks veracity because its effectiveness cannot be demonstrated under laboratory conditions, but it recognizes the value of scientific and clinical trials wherever these are applicable, and the need to establish properly organized training courses for future therapists.

Most of the alternative therapies can prove useful in cases of hypertension, either in helping to reduce it in a direct sense, or in combating adverse factors such as stress, high blood-fat levels, alcohol and tobacco withdrawal symptoms, and high body weight. We have already looked at relaxation methods and hypnotherapy; in this final chapter, we will see what naturopathy, herbal medicine, homoeopathy, and acupuncture have to offer.

Naturopathy

Naturopathic medicine is a complete and distinct form of medicine which concentrates upon the body's inherent capacity for self-healing and self-repair. Its aim is to create suitable conditions for this to take place. The name 'naturopathy' has been used since the turn of the century, but the philosophy underlying the system and many of its methods date back to at least 400 BC and were practised by Hippocrates.

There are three basic tenets of naturopathy:

(1) Only nature heals. It does so by the life force re-establishing harmony and balance, provided we make this possible.
(2) Disease results from the body's attempt to remove impediments to the normal working of its tissues and organs. These impediments are classified into three types, chemical, mechanical, and psychological. Chemical problems refer to aspects of the body's biochemistry. i.e. poor nutrition, inefficient excretion of waste matter through the bowels, kidneys, lungs, skin etc.

Mechanical problems responsible for ill-health include stiff joints, weak or tense muscles, bad posture, and misalignment of the spinal vertebrae, leading to musculoskeletal and nervous system ailments.

The implication of this latter point is wide. Misaligned vertebrae can affect the spinal cord, messages it carries between the brain and the rest of the body, and the parasympathetic and sympathetic ganglia or nerve centres controlling the autonomic nervous system and thereby factors such as the contraction and expansion of blood vessels, the blood pressure etc.

Psychological problems include all the possible adverse effects of stress, anxiety, depression from whatever cause, upon the body and its organs.

(3) The third tenet of naturopathy has already been explained in the discussion about the principal differences between the orthodox and alternative approaches to health and disease. That is, that disease arises from disharmony between body, mind and spirit, and affects the whole body regardless of the fact that overt symptoms may suggest that simply one organ is diseased.

The individuality of each person is regarded as highly important, and the nature of that individuality is held to be partly responsible for his or her health. Each of us possesses certain strengths and weaknesses, and reacts differently under strain. This is why naturopathic practitioners take carefully detailed case histories, and attach considerable importance to inherited defects, the possibility of pre-birth trauma, and the individual's environment.

During a consultation, discussion is followed by a physical examination and relevant biochemical investigations of, for example, urine, blood, sputum (phlegm), secretions etc. Once a diagnosis is reached in the light of all the information gained, the naturopath sets out to decide how best the patient can be helped to help him- or herself.

In dealing with a case of high blood pressure, special importance would be attached to past medical history, health/causes of death of parents and/or close relatives, the state of the heart and circulatory system, the function of the autonomic nervous system, and present/recent stresses, strains, emotional problems and social habits.

Treatment would focus upon diet and weight control along the lines discussed in Chapter 5; advice would be given regarding smoking and alcohol consumption with, perhaps, referral to an acupuncturist or hypnotherapist if extra help were required. Many naturopaths favour fasting as a means of treatment, and this may be suggested, and carried out, with the patient's co-operation, under the therapist's guidance.

Relaxation techniques and exercise regimens would be recommended, perhaps in combination with therapeutic massage. Advice would be given about poor posture, and how it could be rectified. Many naturopathic practitioners practise other forms of alternative medicine in addition to their own. Those skilled in osteopathy might treat spinal misalignment personally, while others would refer their patient to another therapist.

While drugs are regarded essentially as undesirable toxins, no patient would be told by an experienced naturopath to cease taking prescribed medication forthwith. Herbal remedies and dietary supplements compatible with current treatment may well be recommended, but the aim of naturopathic practitioners is to ease the body into a state of health so that, in so far as it is possible, drugs either become unnecessary or can be utilized in smaller doses.

Herbal medicine

Herbal medicine — or, to give it the name many practitioners favour, medical herbalism — is at first difficult to equate with the concept of complementary or alternative medicine. So naturally and imperceptibly has this age-old form of medical practice given rise to current pharmaceutical science and industry that the temptation arises to regard it simply as the worthy but anachronistic precursor of modern drug therapy.

This view is, in fact, grossly unjust to the art and science of medical herbalism which flourishes, and will continue to flourish, as a major and significant form of complementary medicine in its own right. That its foundations are rooted in the earliest attempts to combat disease needs no emphasis here. Certainly, modern pharmacy owes an incalculable debt to the wisdom and expertise of herbal practitioners throughout history; but the fact that medical herbalism has continued to offer enormous benefits to the sick in every race is indisputable.

At a scientific level, herbal preparations can be seen as a source of the essential vitamins, minerals and trace elements needed to promote health and combat disease. At a more comprehensive level, the medicinal substances used by practitioners, culled as they are from whole, living plants, contain within them a complete range of active ingredients co-existing in a harmonious and natural state. According to medical herbalists, it is the state of balance inherent in herbal remedies, as much as the constituents themselves, that is responsible for their curative properties.

Medical herbalists take stock of a patient's presenting symptoms, but attach more importance to his/her overall state of integrated balance and harmony. Their aim is to identify underlying imbalances in the various bodily and psychological systems, to reach a diagnosis, and to treat the whole person by restoring him/her to a state of equilibrium. This explains why different remedies may be employed to treat the same condition in different patients; for, like other complementary therapists, medical herbalists aim at treating the complete person as an individual being.

Practitioners of herbal medicine oppose the extraction of a single, active element from a medicinal plant. They view this strategy as highly conducive to the production of adverse side-effects — an opinion borne out by many recipients of orthodox medicine. Digoxin, for example, prescribed for heart failure, can have serious side-effects when used as a drug. Foxglove extract, by contrast, contains within it a range of natural ingredients which combat heart failure yet, when prescribed judiciously by a competent herbalist, are less inclined to cause adverse reactions.

Herbal remedies for self-administration abound, and are easily accessible, yet they should be taken in strict accordance with the instructions provided. They are no more a 'panacea for all ills' than are vitamins, minerals and other natural supplements, and since they are sufficiently potent to relieve, and often cure, diseases, it follows that their misuse can result in serious consequences.

Most medical herbalists emphasize the importance of consulting a qualified practitioner about all but the most trivial ailments. Treatment for high blood pressure would be aimed in the first instance at the underlying problem of small blood vessel constriction and disease, accompanied by advice about lifestyle changes, stress reduction, exercise, and diet.

Likely remedies would be those with vasodilatory effect, i.e. those capable of relaxing the narrowed walls of the peripheral blood vessels. Important examples include limeflowers, hawthorn and garlic, because of their ability to improve the circulation and tissue oxygenation. These may be prescribed in combination with diuretic herbs, such as parsley, celery, dandelion leaves, wild carrot, and asparagus; and natural relaxants, such as rosemary, lavender, lemon balm, chamomile, and catmint. Substantial falls in blood pressure are often obtained by these measures.

Homoeopathy

Homoeopathy as a system of medicine originated in the research of Dr Samuel Hahnemann, an eighteenth century German physician and chemist. Two prime factors motivated his search for an alternative method of treating patients. The first was his dissatisfaction with orthodox medicine's tendency to treat symptoms rather than patients as individuals. The second was his dislike of the barbarous treatment methods then in fashion. Bleeding, purging, and powerful emetics (to provoke vomiting), stimulants and sedatives were all commonly employed, together with surgery which as yet knew the benefits of neither anaesthesia nor hygiene.

Like naturopathic practitioners, Hahnemann believed in the body's ability to heal itself, and regarded symptoms as evidence of attempts to put that healing ability into practice. In his famous work, *The Organon Of Rational Healing* (1810), he described the vital force which he held responsible for the body's natural healing processes. Again in common with naturopathic philosophy, he was convinced that disease resulted from inner disharmony, and believed that treatment should aim at restoring balance between the physical, mental, and spiritual aspects of human nature.

Biochemistry was one of Hahnemann's particular interests. Using a wide range of natural remedies derived from animal, plant and mineral origins, and himself as guinea pig, he rediscovered a principle of medicine whose validity had been recognized since the time of Hippocrates. This principle states that 'like cures like'.

He started by experimenting with currently used drugs, the difference being that in taking them himself he was using them on a healthy rather than on a sick person.

He discovered that the substances he took produced the symptoms he would have expected had he been suffering from the illness they were normally employed to cure. Quinine, used for malaria, was a case in point. He took sizeable doses for two days, and found that his extremities grew cold; than he became sleepy and exhausted; that his pulse raced, and that he experienced palpitations. He felt extremely anxious, trembled all over, his head throbbed, his face grew flushed and he felt extremely thirsty. Having had malaria earlier in life, he was able to confirm the effects of the quinine to resemble those of the illness very closely.

He concluded from this that quinine overpowered malarial fever by creating a fever of its own, and that the symptoms of the illness were not evidence of the disease itself but of the body's resistance to it. Using both himself and healthy volunteer subjects to discover whether this principle would be borne out in other instances, he was eventually able to confirm that a drug which produced certain symptoms in healthy people was the drug of choice to treat those symptoms when patients became ill.

Just as vaccination with, for example, a tiny quantity of tetanus toxoid causes the immune defence system to produce antibodies against further encounters with the tetanus bacteria, so homoeopathic remedies stimulate the body's inherent healing capacity. Hahnemann soon discovered, too, that the smaller the dose, the greater the effect. Various theories have been put forward to account for this apparent anomaly; and the explanation now seems to lie in the method used in preparing the remedies.

'Mother tinctures' — alcoholic extracts of the plant, mineral or other substance used — are made, and repeatedly diluted (i.e. triturated) a hundredfold. The first dilution is termed 1C; the second, 2C, is a hundredth dilution of the first, i.e. the original tincture diluted 10,000 times. The preparation is then 'succussed' i.e. shaken vigorously by hand or machine many times over. It is this process that is believed to 'potentize' the remedy being prepared, probably by increasing the molecular energy of the active substances it contains. What the patient finally receives is the active substance in a very low concentration but in a state of high energy.

In addition to taking a formal case history, homoeopathic practitioners ask their patients many questions that can, on face value, seen irrelevant. They might want to know whether the symptoms are more troublesome in cold weather or when milk is taken, or whether the individual likes or fears the dark, loud noises or thunderstorms. Importance is also attached to personality, physical appearance, hair colour, skin colour etc. Homoeopaths need this information in order to match the remedies they use as closely as possible to the person they are treating. This is why the same symptoms, e.g. sneezing, fever, sore throat, in three very different patients may be treated with different remedies, picked in each case to conform to the individual as a whole person. Similarly, the same remedy may be selected to treat widely differing symptoms in patients of similar types.

The range of possible remedies for a problem such as high blood pressure is, therefore, wide, but may include NAJA (Naja Naja Naja) for heart failure and/or palpitations; GELS (Gelsemium) for dizzy spells; TAB (Tabacum) for early morning headaches); LYC (Lycopodium Clavatum) for swollen ankles associated with heart failure; PULS (Pulsatilla) to aid weight reduction; and ACON (Aconitum Napellus), SPONG (Spongia Tosta), HEP (Hepar Sulphur) or CALC (Calcarea Ostrearum) for tension and anxiety.

Like herbal medicines, homoeopathic remedies for serious conditions such as high blood pressure are better prescribed by a qualified practitioner than used for self-treatment.

Acupuncture

The origins of acupuncture are uncertain, but evidence exists that it was practised in China as long ago as the third millenium BC. Huan Ti, who became Emperor of China and was known as the Father of Acupuncture, worked together with his personal physician Ch'i Po to establish the principles of anatomy, health, and disease upon which this medical art is based. Huan Ti described his findings in *Nei Ching* (the Yellow Emperor's Classic of Internal Medicine), a book that remained the definitive authority on the subject for many centuries.

Like other forms of holistic medicine, acupuncture sees disease as the result of disharmony, in particular of blockage of the life force, ch'i, which is considered to pass along invisible lines known as meridians running throughout the body. Two great life elements called yin and yang, complementary opposites, remain in a state of balance when a person is healthy, permitting ch'i to flow freely along the meridian lines. But when yin and yang become unbalanced, through inherent weakness, stress, the effects of toxins and other adverse factors, ch'i's flow is impeded, giving rise to the symptoms of illness.

Yin and yang are elements in all traditional Eastern philosphies. They are polar opposites, present in all things, and can be discerned throughout nature at every juncture. Examples include the male and female principles, coldness and heat, wetness and dryness, hardness and softness, dominance and receptivity, activity and passivity, positive and negative, light and darkness, day and night.

Like other comparable systems, yin and yang exist in a state of mutual but dynamic equilibrium, which exists as a coherent and live 'whole', elements of each principle fluctuating while the complete system remains in a state of balance. When adverse factors such as those mentioned above upset the state of equilibrium, allowing either yin or yang to hold sway over the other, the effects are felt at the level of the life force, and the living organism suffers accordingly.

The object of an acupuncturist is to identify the underlying problem and to treat it by removing the obstruction to ch'i's free flow, thereby restoring harmony and health. He or she takes a detailed case history, examines the patient, considers the relevant organs in terms of their yin and yang characteristics, determines the meridian lines involved, and completes the diagnosis by taking the pulses at each wrist — a far more complex and detailed enterprise than pulse examination in conventional medicine.

Treatment consists of stimulating certain high energy points (i.e. acupuncture points) along the meridian lines by means of needles, heat (moxibustion), and/or modern innovations such as electromagnetic energy, polarized light, low power lasers and tuning forks vibrating at a certain required resonance. Its effect is to unblock the clogged meridian(s) and restore yin and yang to harmonious and integrated balance.

Acupuncture was first heard of in Europe in the seventeenth century, when missionaries from China told of its practice on their return to the West. A few Chinese specialists practised it in the UK in the early part of this century, but it did not become known to the general public until the late 1950s. With the great growth of interest in alternative medicine in the 1960s and 1970s, acupuncture flourished and became widely practised.

Its frequent successes naturally caused much controversy. Initially, most orthodox doctors were highly sceptical, and attributed cures to that well-known panacea for many ills, the placebo effect. Later, research was carried out on volunteers under scientifically controlled conditions, and the existence of both meridican lines and acupuncture supported by considerable evidence.

Acupuncture is now practised in Britain by both medically qualified doctors and by lay therapists. Not all practitioners necessarily subscribe — or even understand — the basic Chinese philosophy involving ch'i, yin and yang; but results continue to justify the growing popularity of this form of alternative medicine.

It can help in cases of hypertension by reducing the blood pressure reading, although the beneficial effects often require 'top up' treatment sessions if they are to be maintained. It can help withdrawal symptoms from both tobacco and alcohol, and has permitted many longtime smokers to give up the habit. Beyond doubt, acupuncture has a harmonizing and energizing effect on mind and body, and can help food cravings in overweight people as well as anxiety and tension.

Useful addresses

The British Naturopathic and Osteopathic Association, Frazer House, 6 Netherhall Gardens, London NW3; tel. (071) 435 8728.

National Institute of Medical Herbalists, P.O. Box 3, Winchester, Hants; tel. (0962) 68776.

Society of Homoeopaths, 2 Artizan Road, Northampton NN1 4HU; tel. (0604) 21400.

British Acupuncture Association and Register, 34 Alderney Street, London SW1V 4EU; tel. (071) 834 1012.

Traditional Acupuncture Society, 11 Grange Park, Stratford upon Avon, Warwickshire CV37 6XH; tel. (0789) 298798.

National Council of Psychotherapists and Hypnotherapists, 1 Clovelly Road, Ealing, London W5.

Professional associations outside the UK

Outside the UK, you should be able to obtain addresses from the Yellow Pages, but here are some suggestions for the USA and Australia:

American Association of Naturopathic Physicians
900 Madison Street, Seattle, WA 98104 (206 328-7971)

Traditional Acupuncture Foundation
American City Building, Columbia, MD 21044

International Foundation for Homeopathy
2366 Eastlake East, No. 301, Seattle, WA 98102 (206 324-8230)

Australian Natural Therapeutic Association
31 Victoria Street, Fitzroy, Melbourne

Australian Traditional Medicine Society
Rozelle, Victoria

Australian Homoeopathic Association
c/o 16a Edward Street, Gordon, NSW 2027

National Herbalists Association of Australia
27 Leith Street, Cooparoo, Queensland 4151

Index

ACE inhibitor drugs, 15-16,
   54-5
acupuncture, 113, 114, 121-3
adrenergic neurone blocking
   drugs, 16-17
age, 34-5
alcohol, 49, 68, 70, 109-12
alpha blockers, 17, 55
alpha-beta blockers, 17, 55
alternative treatments, 12, 59,
   113-23
amino acids, 79-80, 85-6
angina, 44-5
antihypertensive drugs, 11-22,
   48-9, 51-2, 53-5
arteries, 42-3, 90
atherosclerosis, 38, 40, 41-3
autonomic nervous system,
   96-7

beta blockers, 14, 48-9, 53-4
biofeedback training, 100-3
bioflavonoids, 83
blood
   clotting, 42
   red cells, 32-3
   thickness, 29, 32-3
   see also cholesterol levels
blood pressure

controlling, 12, 28-30, 37,
   50-2
definition, 23
function of, 27
high see hypertension
low, 27
measuring, 7, 27-8, 33-4
nature of, 26
brain damage, 107, 110

caffeine, 68
calcium, 84
calcium antagonist drugs, 15,
   54
calorie intake, 69, 75
cancer, 66, 105
carbohydrates, 64-5
carbon monoxide, 107
carnitine, 79-80
chemoreceptor depressant
   drugs, 17
cholesterol levels, 13, 33, 45
   diet to reduce, 72-4
cigarettes see smoking
circulation, 23-6, 28-9, 77-82
claudication, 90
CNS depressant drugs, 16
coffee, 68
CoQ (coenzyme Q), 82

coronary heart disease, 38, 43-6, 89-90

dairy products, 64, 66, 69
death rate, 46, 61
diabetes, 90-1
diet, 43, 60-74
dietary supplements, 76-86
diuretics, 13-14, 18-19, 53
doctor–patient relationship, 52-3
drinks, 68
drug treatments, 11-22, 48-55, 59
    dosages, 20, 50-2
    problems with, 11-13
    side-effects, 11, 13-17, 19, 20
    taking medication, 17-20
drugs causing hypertension, 33

elderly people, 18, 49-50, 94-5, 111
environmental influences, 35-6
EPA (eicosapentaenoic acid), 80-1
evening primrose oil, 81-2, 85
exercise, 87-95

familial hypercholesterol-aemia, 72
fat in diet, 64, 67-8, 69, 74
fatty acids, 67-8, 80-1, 85
fibre, 64, 65-6, 70
fish, 66, 69
fish oil supplements, 80-1
fruit and vegetables, 65, 69

ganglion blocker drugs, 17

GLA (gammalinolenic acid), 81-2, 85
glandular malfunction, 32
grains, 65, 66, 67

health and vitality diet, 63-8
heart
    attacks, 45-6
    disease, 38, 43-6, 91
    failure, 38-9
herbalism, 113, 117-19
histidine, 80
homoeopathy, 113, 119-21
human growth hormone (HGH), 85
hypertension, 7, 27
    causes, 31-3
    definition, 30-1
    diet to reduce, 69-72
    dietary supplements for, 77-82
    and health problems, 37-46
    malignant, 45-6, 50
    mild and moderate, 48-50, 50-2
    risk factors, 34-6, 37, 104-5
    screening for, 33-4
    treatment, 37, 47-55
        see also alternative treatments; drug treatments
hyperlipidaemia, 72-3
hypnotherapy, 101, 108-9
hypoglycaemia, 65

immune system, 43, 114

kidney failure, 38, 39-40

life expectancy, 37, 46
lifestyle, 7, 11, 48

magnesium, 84
malignant hypertension *see*
　hypertension
malnutrition, 63, 77
meat, 66, 69
meditation, 100, 102
men, 35
myocardial infarction, 45

narrowing of aorta, 32
natural treatments *see*
　alternative treatments
naturopathy, 115-17
nephrotic syndrome, 73
nervous system, 96-7, 110
neuromuscular relaxation,
　99-100
nicotine, 106-7

obesity, 14, 22, 36, 61, 74-5
oils, cooking, 67-8
orthodox treatments, 11-13,
　114-15
osteoporosis, 90

parasympathetic nervous
　system, 97-8
peripheral vascular disorders,
　38, 105
placebo effect, 18
polycythaemia, 32-3
polyunsaturated fats, 67-8, 74
potassium, 13, 18, 69
pregnancy, 32
primary hypertriglycerid-
　aemia, 72
processed foods, 63, 64, 77
progressive muscular
　relaxation, 99-100, 102
protein, 66-7
pulse rates and exercise, 93-4

pulses, 65, 66, 67

racial differences, 35-6
reflexology, 113
relaxation techniques, 96-103
rauwolfia alkaloid drugs, 20-1
renal disease, 31-2, *see also*
　kidney failure

salt intake, 36, 64, 69
saturated fats, 64, 66, 67-8,
　74, 85
selenium, 78-9
senile dementia, 41
sex differences, 35, 49, 105-6
sleep, 91
smoking, 22, 49, 104-9
sport, 45
　see also exercise
stepped care treatment, 50-2
stress, 34, 77, 82-4, 89, 96
strokes, 38, 40-1
sugar intake, 64, 65
swimming, 88, 92
sympathetic nervous system,
　96-8

taurine, 80
tea, 68
transient ischaemic attacks,
　40-1

vasodilator drugs, 14-15, 54
vitality, 63-8
vitamin B, 83-4
vitamin C, 82-3, 106
vitamin E, 78-9

walking, 88, 92
water pills *see* diuretics
weight control, 36, 60-1, 69,

74-5, 85-6
see also obesity
whole foods, 61-72
definition, 62-3
and public attitudes, 61-2

women, 35, 46, 49, 105-6

yoga, 102

zinc, 84